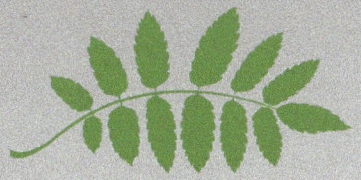

WEST END ORGANIX

Ageless Beauty, Organic Health

Look and feel younger and healthier with our natural remedies products!

www.WestEndOrganix.com

Discount: 10% off of your order - Code *WEO2021*

Pump it up Magazine

TABLE OF CONTENTS

EDITORIAL
Page 5

YULIA
Smooth Jazz Pianist
From Russia With A Sign of Love!

6

2022! HERE WE GLOW
Brain Food:
Eat Yourself Smart!
GET FIT in 21 days!
Try our 4 Weeks
Exercice Plan

MUSIC
Top Independent Music Artists -
New Weekly Top 20 Charts
on PIUMP RADIO

10

STYLE
New Trends for 2022

BEAUTY
New Trends for 2022

18

TOP TIPS
Musician Social
Media Strategy

CINEMA
Books to Movies and T.V.
in 2022

26

HUMANITARIAN AWARENESS
How Amazing it is ...When I reflect ....
Mind and Mumbling
by Alan Laird

Pump it up
MAGAZINE

PUMP IT UP MAGAZINE

LINKS

WEBSITE
www.pumpitupmagazine.com

FACEBOOK
www.facebook.com/pumpitupmagazine

TWITTER
www.twitter.com/pumpitupmag

SOUNDCLOUD
www.soundcloud.com/pumpitupmagazine

INSTAGRAM
pumpitupmagazine

PINTEREST
www.pinterest.com/pumpitupmagazine

PUMP IT UP MAGAZINE
30721 Russell Ranch Road
Suite 140
Westlake Village,
California 91362
United States
www.pumpitupmagazine.com
info@pumpitupmagazine.com
Tel : (001) (877)841 – 7414 (toll free number)

EDITORIAL

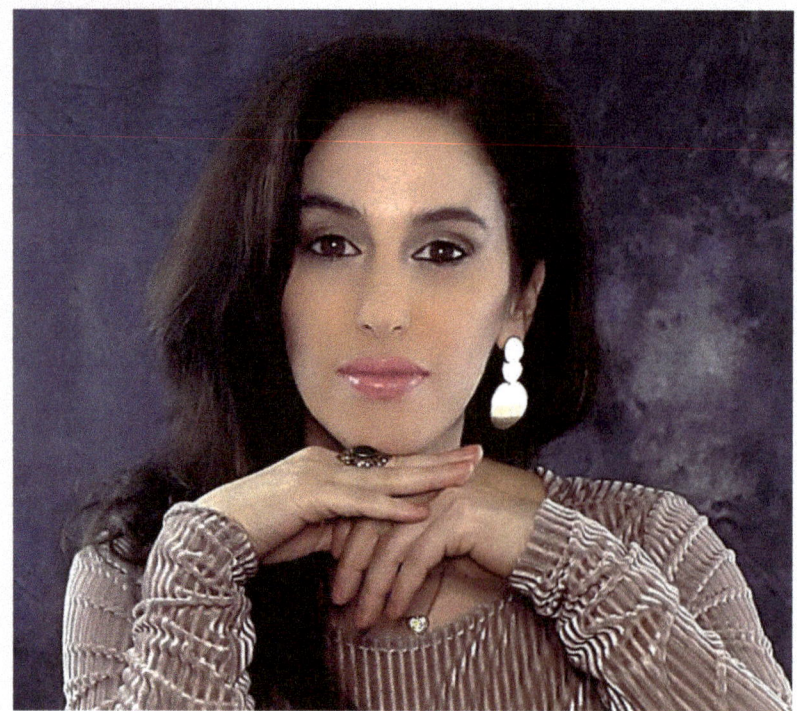

Greetings and Happy New Year readers!

We'll have you made your New Years resolution? Whatever your New Years' resolution is, we here at Pump it up Magazine wish you the best!

On the cover of this issue is the talented Russian-born smooth jazz pianist/composer Yulia! What a talent! Her new single " Sign of Love" has already graced the Digital Radio Tracker chart in the top 100 and she continues to wow everyone with her clever and eclectic style. Truly is a master of the keyboard Don't forget to read her interview in the pages ahead.

Looking to get fit (or shall I say more fit) in 2022? Check out Pump It Magazines 4 week workout plan Let's Glow!

Ready for the next Viral Fashion trends that will take over this year and beyond?
Check out the fashion page on page 14.
Also our beauty trends this year are taking us to some of the leading products to give you that 2022 glow from head to toe!

And check out our top indie artists this year!
Mitchell Coleman Jr and his smash single " Glide" A Funk/Fusion/Smooth Jazz cover of the popular track by the group " Pleasure"
Michael B Sutton " Bandaid for a Broken Heart" is A track sure to do more than patch up a broken heart Aneessa " Miles Away" a Smooth Madonna cover

Saint Jaimz: This CEO and Mogul is bringing back the iconic sound of 90's R&B. All that soul and hear-filled lyrics that we missed Saint Jaimz will
warm your heart and soul as he takes you back to the good ol days when R&B was exactly what is says

Please don't forget to check out Pump It Up Magazine Radio's Smooth Jazz show every Friday Morning and Friday evening with DJ Bernie C.

And some Hip Hop and Urban gems from Grandmixer GMS .
All on Pump It Up Magazine Radio

In our top tips section, we want to share with you more strategies to improve your Social Media presence and branding.

Finally, as this New Year begins we want to invite your attention to our monthly Humanitarian Awareness pages.

This month is about mental health.

The past two years have had devastating effects on the mental health of many.

Anxiety, Depression, OCD, suicides have gone up and we pray that those suffering may find solace in the following articles and pages.

It has taken a toll on children as well as adults.

Entrepreneur, author, and artist Alan Laird, Asks us to pause and reflect upon….

Best of life, health and love to all

Anissa and Michael B. Sutton

CONTRIBUTORS

EDITOR IN CHIEF
GRAPHIC DESIGNER
Anissa B. Sutton

ENTERTAINMENT
Michael B. Sutton
A. Scott Galloway
Sarah Kaye

LIFESTYLE
Tiffani Sutton

AWARENESS
Alan Laird

MARKETING
Grace Rose
Robert Steward
Carter Kaya

PARTNERS

Editions L.A.
www.editions-la.com

The Sound Of L.A.
www.thesoundofla.com

Info Music
www.infomusic.fr

Delit Face
www.DelitFace.com

L.A. Unlimited
www.launlimitedinc.com

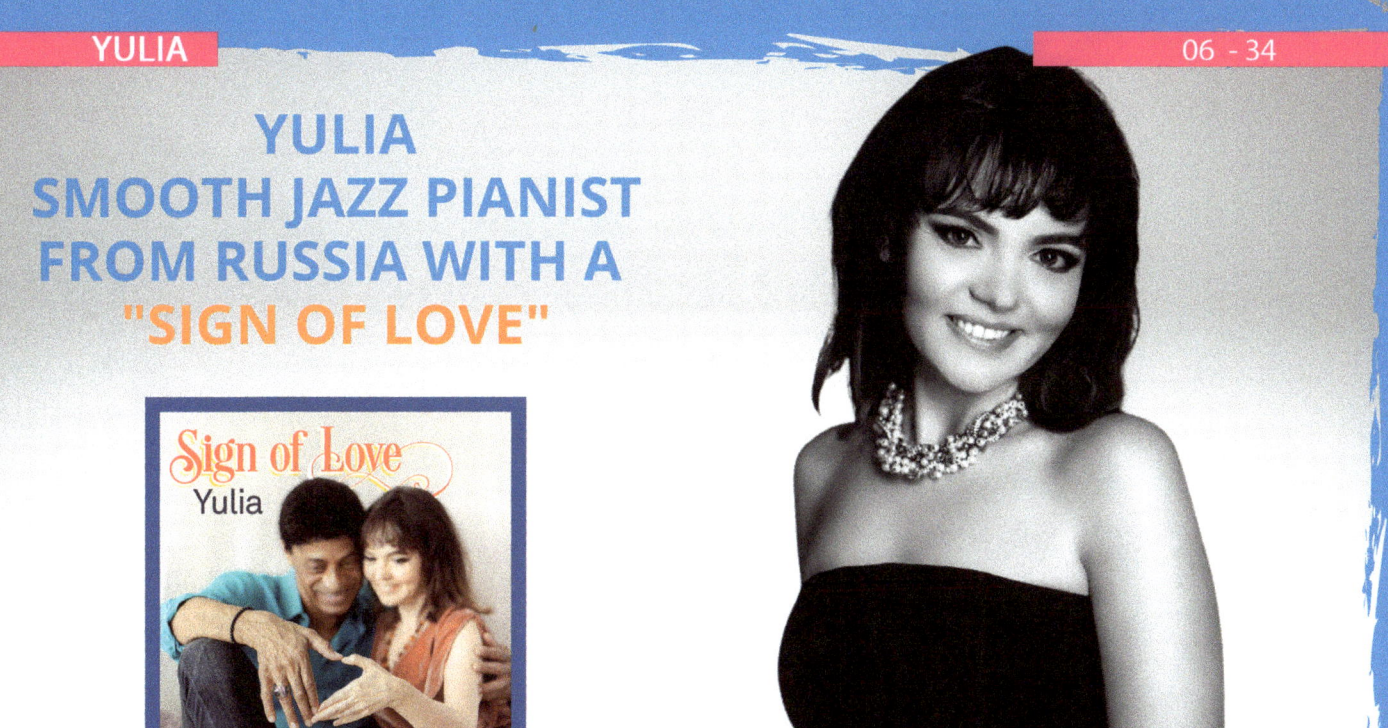

YULIA
SMOOTH JAZZ PIANIST FROM RUSSIA WITH A "SIGN OF LOVE"

The 2021 Best original music composer at the Nieves International Christian Film festival, "Yulia," has stood out to be one of the best jazz music composers since her debut back in 2016.

The ingenious gifted artist has composed several jazz pieces over a couple of years that are unlike, and she is not yet to stop. Yulia released her new solo dubbed "Sign of Love"

"Sign of Love" features a seamless flow of melodies that are just going to interact with its listeners. Most of the extraordinary music that Yulia has released has crossed the borders of jazz music into the universal realm of religion, society and has caused a positive change in so many ways.

With the title of her single being a sign that is popular with everyone, you can't doubt that this will be a force in jazz music.

In her beautiful jazzy and remarkably catchy single "Perfect Love," that is already available for streaming, Yulia improvised with the rhythm of the whole track. Made with a lot of creativity, one would have thought that no other music comes close to the incredible level of telepathic communication and improvisatory genius. However, the prodigy has come to defy all the beliefs with her new single.

"Sign of Love" is a whole conversation, a song written for her soulmate, that all lovers of jazz music will enjoy for the upcoming festive season, and it will indeed speak to you at some point.

Yulia Petrova is generally skilled in composing jazz music with a distinguished level of creativeness. Her blend of different instruments delivers a unique sound with a very firm grip on music theory.

Her musical improvisation will leave you surprised when I listen to her music.
Her kind of jazz fits all moments and occasions.

You can keep up with the latest news from Yulia about her new single by following her social media and streaming platform pages, or using her website: https://www.imyulia.com/

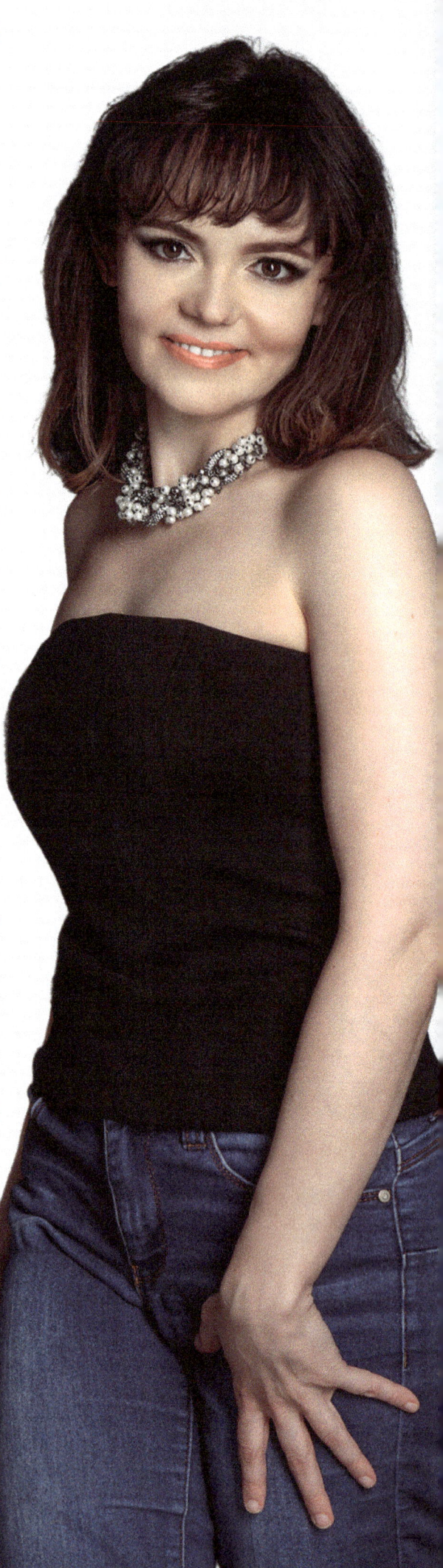

HOW AND WHEN DID MUSIC FIRST COME INTO YOUR LIFE?

YULIA : As I remember myself I loved to sing. I didn't know notes before my age 5 but I think I understood birds that time very well (lol). We had a piano at home and my parents found a piano teacher - and then my more conscious love for music began.

WHAT ARE YOUR EARLIEST RECOLLECTIONS OF JAZZ?

YULIA: During my childhood, jazz music was not so popular. Domestic jazz performers, as a rule, were not prohibited, but harsh criticism of jazz as such was widespread, in the context of criticism of Western culture in general.
The first jazz compositions that began to awaken my interest were compositions by the Arsenal group that I heard in 80s.. In the 90s, jazz festivals began to be held in my city, and I was a grateful listener. Also, the musicians shared recordings of jazz and blues music and that time I could have opportunity to listen to it.

WHAT ADVICE WOULD YOU GIVE TO A YOUNGER JAZZ WRITER?

YULIA: Each composer expresses what he feels inside. In my opinion, it is very important to pass your music through your heart and your thoughts, only then the music will have its own individuality, its own style. My advice is to listen to other musicians, learn from them to understand the language of music, but look for your own words to answer.

HOW IS THE SMOOTH JAZZ SCENE IN RUSSIA COMPARED TO AMERICA?

YULIA: From the beginning of the 90s to the present, a lot has changed. Much more jazz began to sound in Russia, and the number of connoisseurs of this genre is growing as well.

WHO ARE YOUR GREATEST MUSICAL INFLUENCES IN SMOOTH JAZZ?

YULIA: Bob James, George Benson, Marcus Miller, Stanley Clark, Dave Grusin, Andreas Vollenweider..

WHAT ARE YOUR MUSICAL GOALS FOR 2022 AND BEYOND

YULIA: To write, to write and don't stop to write.
God gave me a talent I need to use it and have a joy and bring the joy to others. All the positive energy I use in my music I wish can help people be more positive and feel the blessings that we all have.
Thank you! Best wishes and blessings in 2022!

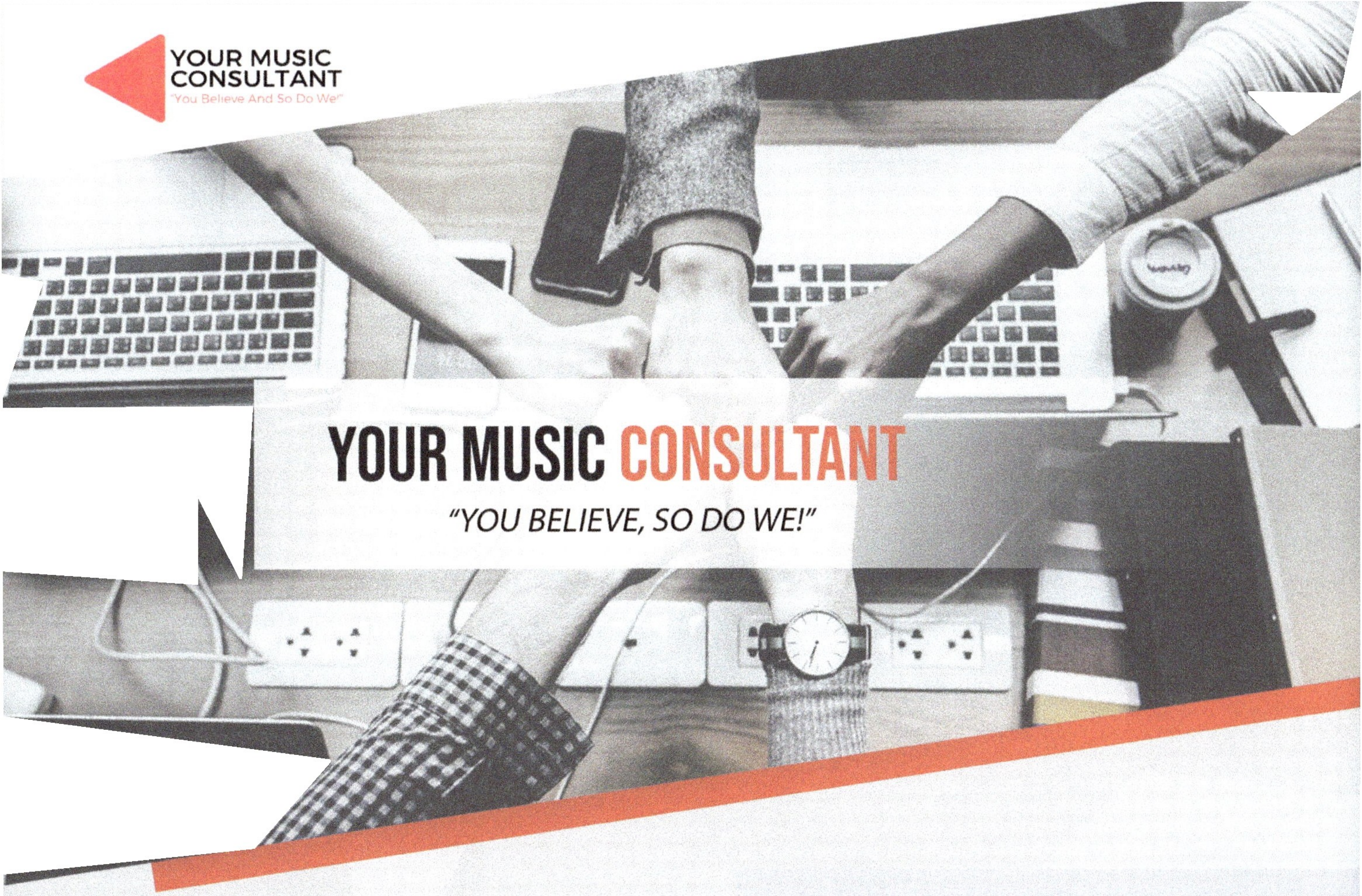

YOUR MUSIC CONSULTANT

"YOU BELIEVE, SO DO WE!"

We Can Help You To Grow Your Business

We are a monthly based service, we put faith in artists who has major potential, believed in them, and who are willing to spend their time and own money to work with us in building a successful music career!

Digital Marketing Services

SOCIAL MEDIA - STREAMING SERVICES - MUSIC DISTRIBUTION - PRESS RELEASE - PRESS DISTRIBUTION - PR

Radio Airplay and TV Commercial

TERRESTRIAL AND DIGITAL RADIO CAMPAIGN AL GENRES EXCEPT HEAVY METAL - CABLE TV AND MAJOR NETWORK COMMERCIAL

Licensing & Booking

CONCERTS, LIVE MUSIC, EVENTS, CLUB NIGHTS - RED CARPETS - FOREIGN LICENSING AND SUB0PUBLISHING

Why Choose Us ?

3 DECADES OF MUSIC BUSINESS EXPERIENCE
Platinium and Gold Records
MOTOWN RECORDS
UNIVERSAL
SONY
CAPITOL RECORDS

WE WORKED WITH:
Kanye West - Jay Z - Stevie Wonder - Michael Jackson - Germaine Jackson Smokey Robinson - Dionne Warwick - Cheryl Lynn - The Originals -

📞 **1-818-514-0038**
(Ext. 1)
Monday - Friday / 9am to 6pm

FIND US :

www.YourMusicConsultant.com
30721 Russell Ranch Road Suite 140 Westlake Village, USA
Email : info@yourmusicconsultant.com

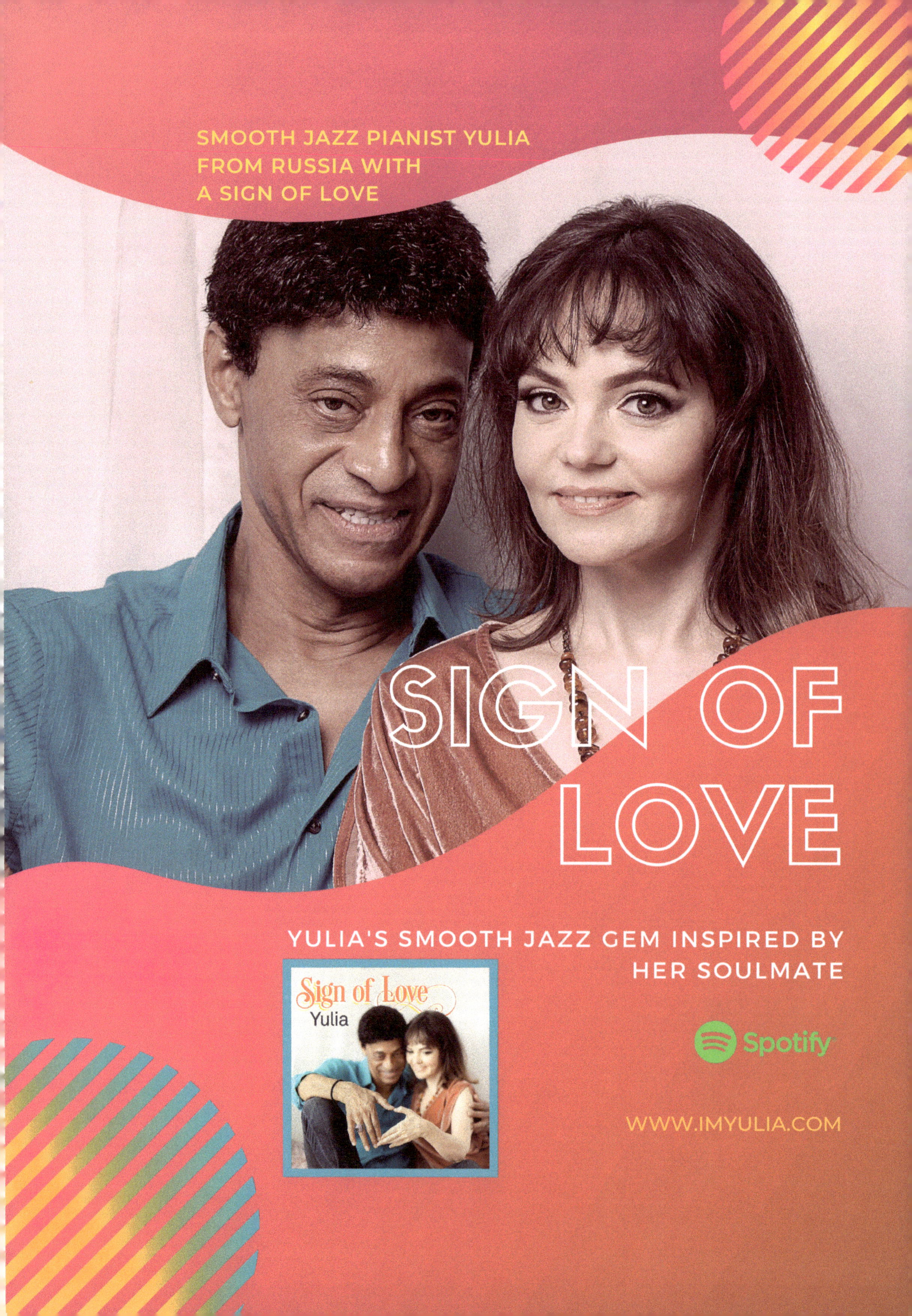

SMOOTH JAZZ PIANIST YULIA FROM RUSSIA WITH A SIGN OF LOVE

SIGN OF LOVE

YULIA'S SMOOTH JAZZ GEM INSPIRED BY HER SOULMATE

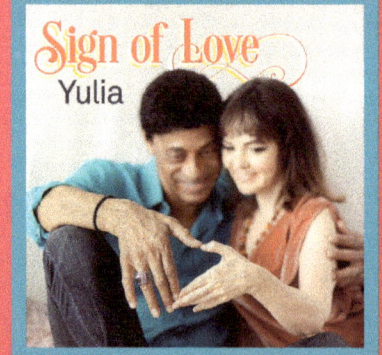

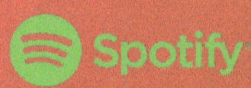

WWW.IMYULIA.COM

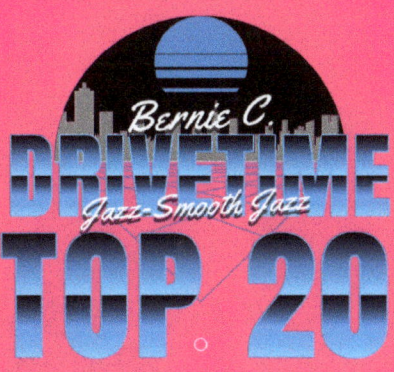

Every Friday Morning 7am-9am (PST) - 10AM-12AM(EST)
Every Friday Evening 7pm-9pm (PST) -10PM-12PM(EST)

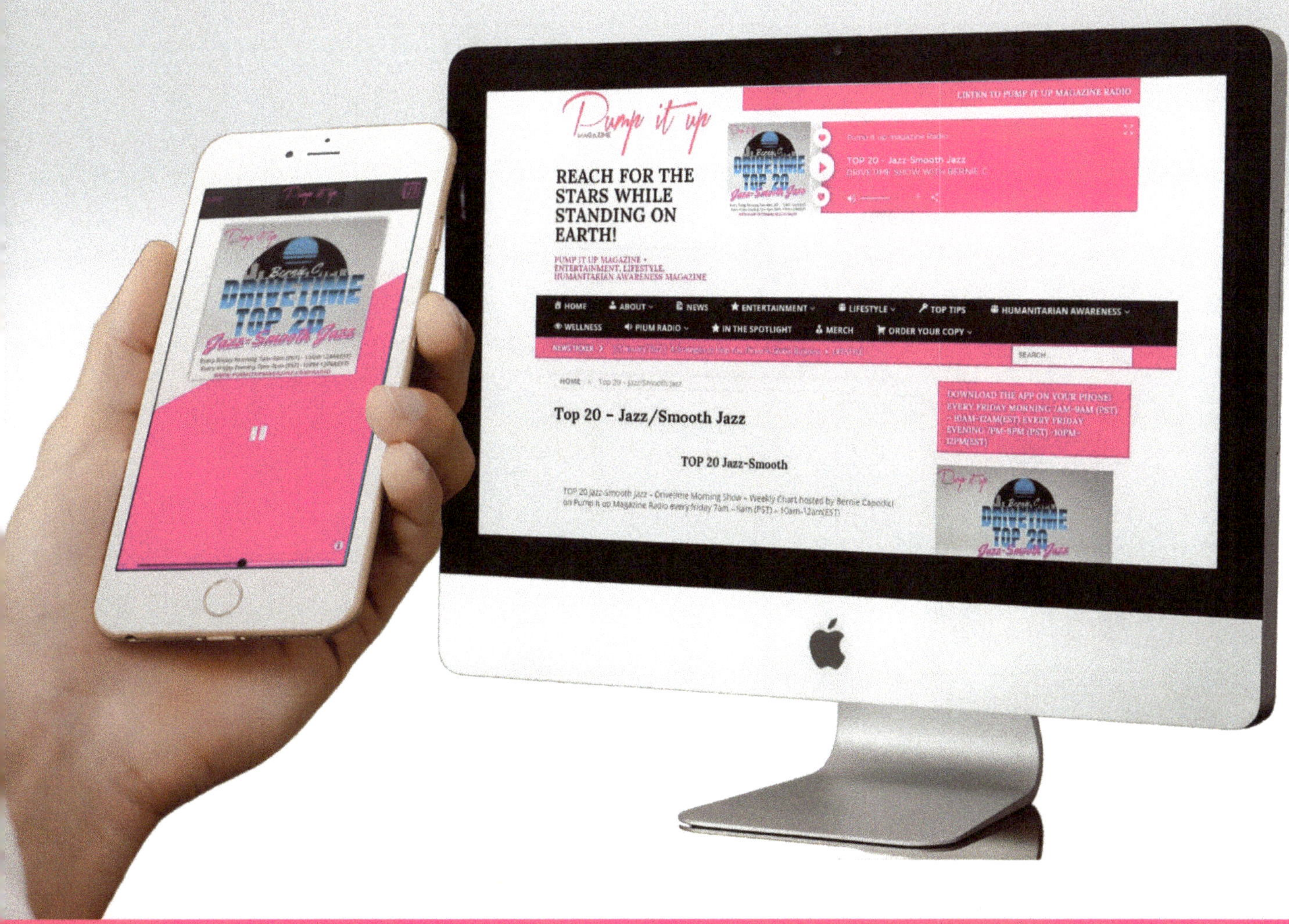

**DOWNLOAD NOW
PUMP IT UP MAGAZINE RADIO APP
ON YOUR PHONE
WWW.PUMPITUPMAGAZINE.COM/RADIO**

EAT YOURSELF SMART
FOOD FOR THE BRAIN

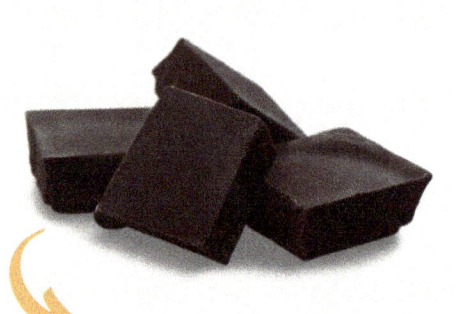

DARK CHOCOLATE

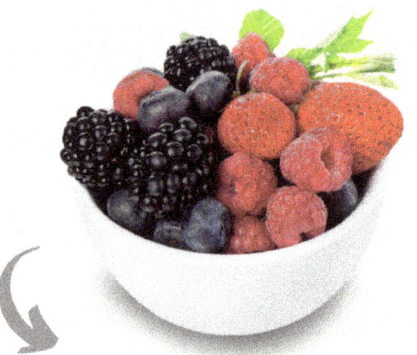

BERRIES

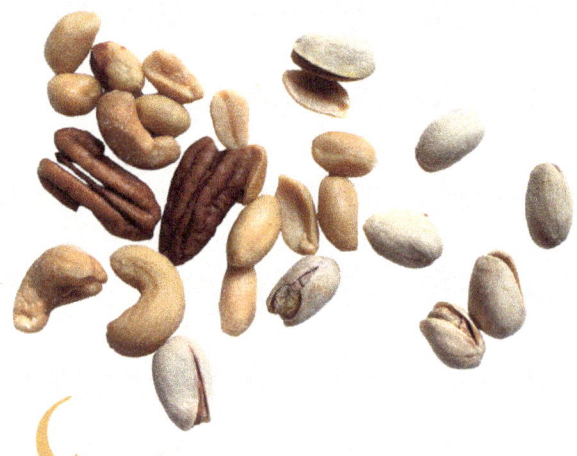

NUTS & SEEDS

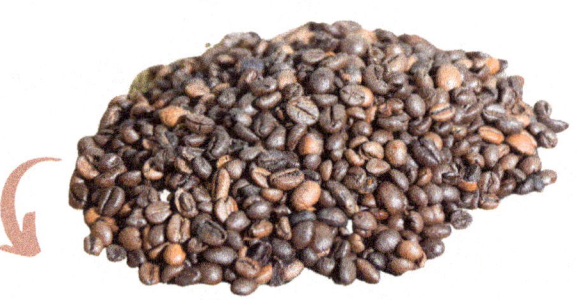

COFFEE

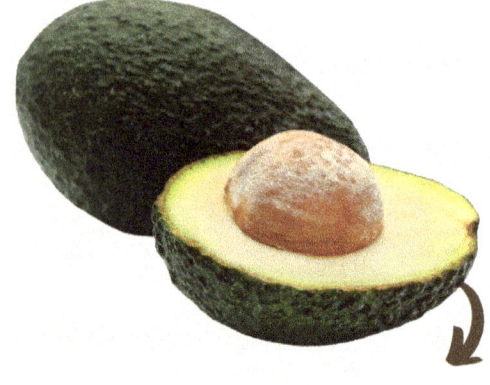

AVOCADOS

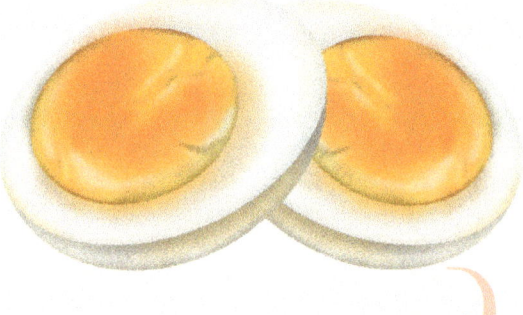

EGGS

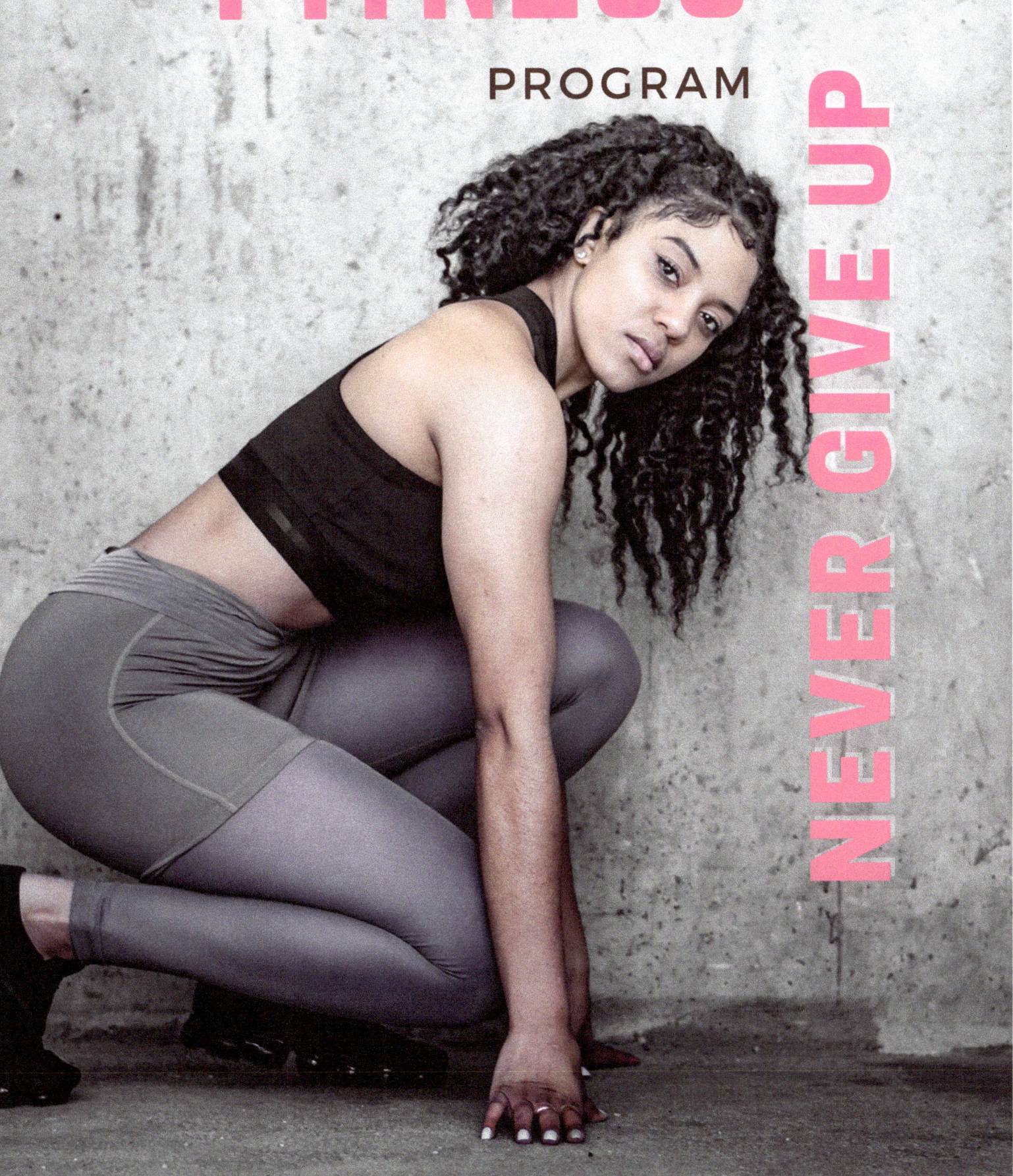

4 WEEKS WORKOUT PLAN

SUN
- 45 jumping jacks
- 15 squats
- 5 jump squats
- 50 Russian twists
- 30 second plank
- 10 standing calf raises
- 5 kneeling pushups
- 30 seconds Superman
- 10 lunges (each leg)
- 40 crunches

MON
- 45 jumping jacks
- 15 squats
- 5 jump squats
- 50 Russian twists
- 30 second plank
- 10 standing calf raises
- 5 kneeling pushups
- 30 seconds Superman
- 10 lunges (each leg)
- 40 crunches

TUES
- 45 jumping jacks
- 15 squats
- 5 jump squats
- 50 Russian twists
- 30 second plank
- 10 standing calf raises
- 5 kneeling pushups
- 30 seconds Superman
- 10 lunges (each leg)
- 40 crunches

WED
- 45 jumping jacks
- 15 squats
- 5 jump squats
- 50 Russian twists
- 30 second plank
- 10 standing calf raises
- 5 kneeling pushups
- 30 seconds Superman
- 10 lunges (each leg)
- 40 crunches

THURS
- 45 jumping jacks
- 15 squats
- 5 jump squats
- 50 Russian twists
- 30 second plank
- 10 standing calf raises
- 5 kneeling pushups
- 30 seconds Superman
- 10 lunges (each leg)
- 40 crunches

FRI
- 45 jumping jacks
- 15 squats
- 5 jump squats
- 50 Russian twists
- 30 second plank
- 10 standing calf raises
- 5 kneeling pushups
- 30 seconds Superman
- 10 lunges (each leg)
- 40 crunches

SAT
- 45 jumping jacks
- 15 squats
- 5 jump squats
- 50 Russian twists
- 30 second plank
- 10 standing calf raises
- 5 kneeling pushups
- 30 seconds Superman
- 10 lunges (each leg)
- 40 crunches

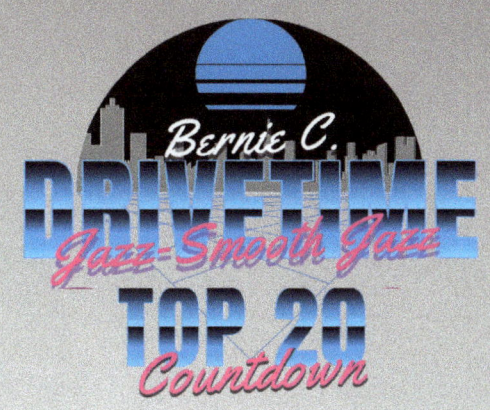

#20 Patric Bradley - Completely Yours
#19 Thom Rotella - She Knows What She Wants
#18 Les Sabler - Esselle's Dance
#17 Phillip "Doc" Martin The Doc Is In The House
Featured Artist Andrew Neu & Rob Zinn - A To Z
#16 Kim Scott f/Althea Rene & Ragen Whitside - I'm Every Woman
#15 Norman Brown - Heart To Heart
#14 Pamela Willams f/ Gerald Albright - Serendipity
#13 Jeff Ryan f/ Adam Hawley - New Day
Featured Artist - Aneessa - Miles Away
#12 Judha Sealy - Stylish
#11 Jazmin Ghent - Get Ready
#10 Richard Smith f/ Richard Elliot
#9 Laid Back - JT Project
Featured Artist - Drivetime - Mysterious Life
#8 Paul Tylor - Straight To The Point
#7 Dave Koz - The Closer We Get
#6 Le Sonic f/ Robert Lee - Any Moment
#5 Gerald Albright - Crazy
Featured Artist - Yulia - A Sign Of Love
#4 Jacob Webb f/ JazminGhent - Nothing Better
#3 Radny Scott f/ Cindy Bradley - Daydreams
#2 Boney James - Sundance
Featured Artist - Michael B. Sutton - Band Aid For A Broken Heart
#1 Phil Denny - Urban Troubadour

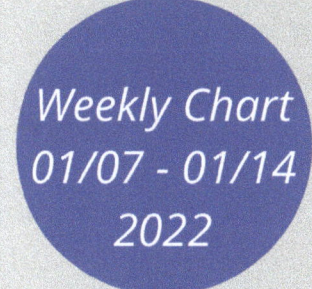

Weekly Chart
01/07 - 01/14
2022

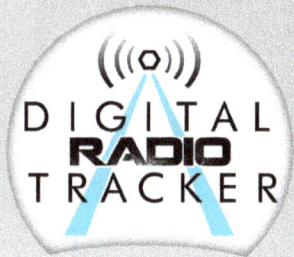

Every Friday Morning 7am-9am (PST) - 10AM-12AM(EST)
Every Friday Evening 7pm-9pm (PST) -10PM-12PM(EST)
WWW.PUMPITUPMAGAZINE.COM/RADIO

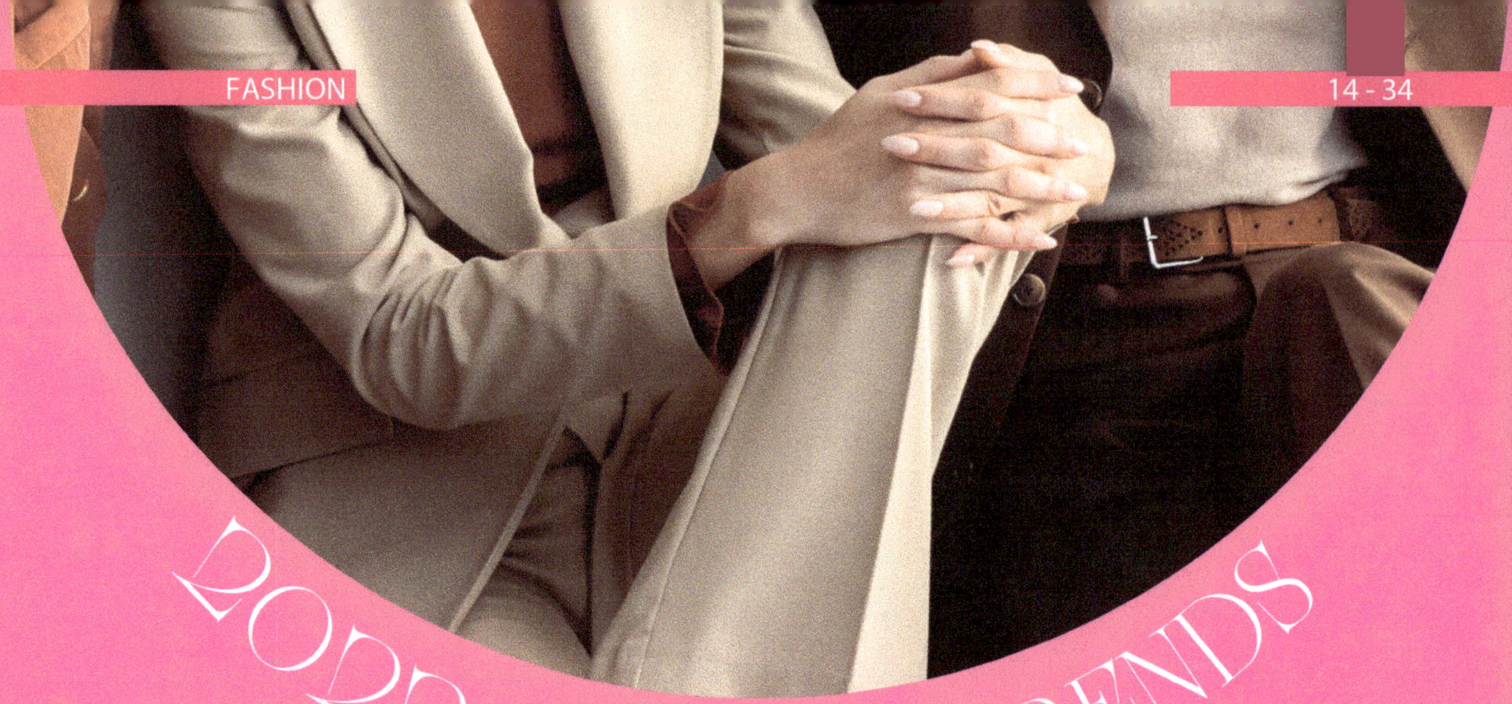

FASHION 14 - 34

2022 FASHION TRENDS

READY FOR THE NEXT VIRAL FASHION TRENDS THAT ARE ABOUT TO TAKE OVER FOR THE YEAR AHEAD? WE ARE EYEING A FRESH SET THAT WE ARE PREDICTING WILL BE EVERYWHERE IN 2022.

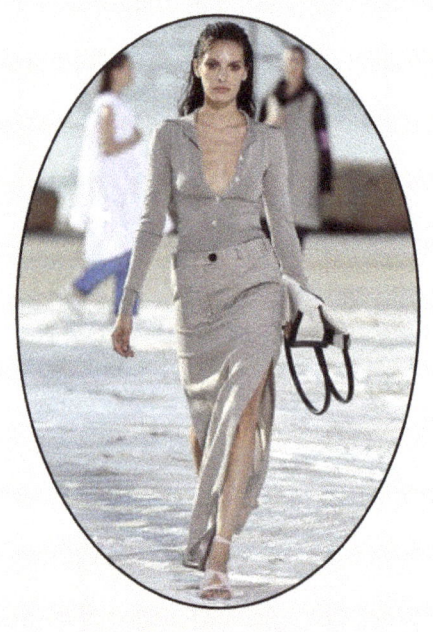 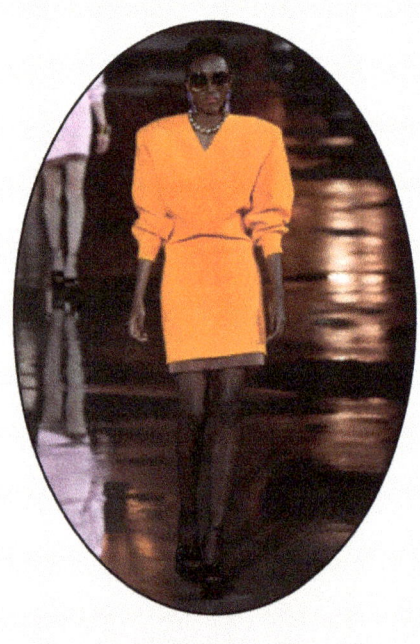 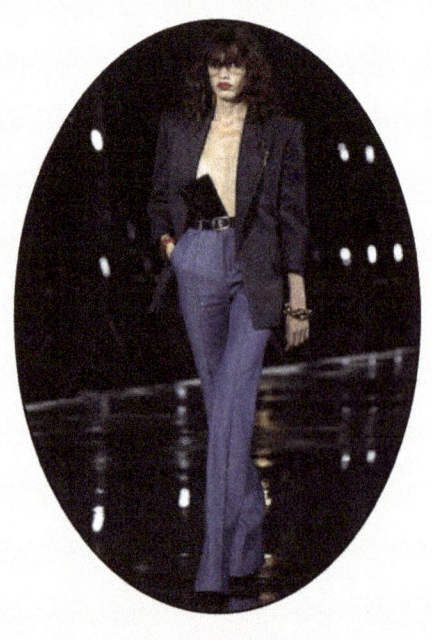

| MAXI HEMLINES | ELECTRIC COLORS | DARK DENIM |

Pump it up Magazine / 14 - 34

VISIT OUR WEBSITE

L.A. UNLIMITED

APPAREL REPRESENTATION
WITHOUT LIMITS...

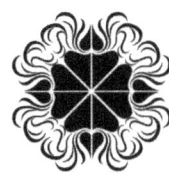

- Corporate Brand Representation
- Brand Identity & Management
- Brand Consulting
- Trade Show Preparation & Participation
- Trunk Shows
- Private Label Sales
- Production Sourcing

L.A. Unlimited & Associates
30765 Pacific Coast Hwy STE 443Malibu, CA 90265

310.882.6432
sales@launlimitedinc.com

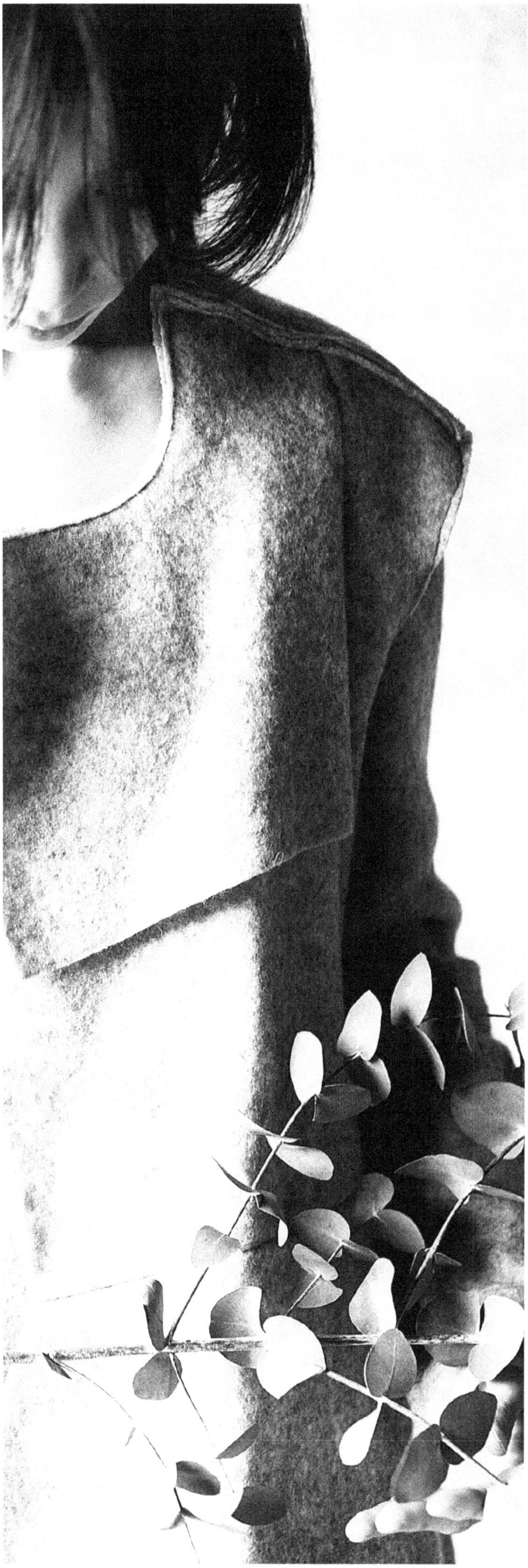

FASHION TRENDS 2022

Ready for the next viral fashion trends that are about to take over for the year ahead? I'm eyeing a fresh set that I'm predicting will be everywhere in 2022. Judging by the S/S 22 runways, there are a number that are primed for adoption amongst the fashion set. But there are already some that we're seeing in circulation that will only get bigger in the coming months. I'm personally buying some of these already and know they have major viral qualities.

So, which ones are the best to add to your closet now? From the color trend that will eclipse neutrals and skin-baring hemlines to the new take on denim for the year ahead and the way fashion people will buy investment pieces, there are plenty to have on your radar. Ahead, the 8 viral fashion trends to know about for 2022 before they blow up.

1. ELECTRIC COLORS

While colors like Kelly green have dominated in the past year, so have neutrals. If you're wondering if you should add some bold shades to your closet, now is definitely the time. Forget low-impact shades, though, because it's bold colors that will soon be all over your feeds.

2. MAXI HEMLINES

One the other end of the spectrum from mini skirts? Maxi hemlines. As I mentioned, there is no middle ground. Consider midi skirts the piece to skip right now because it's all about maxi skirts if you're not into the micro lengths.

3. DARK DENIM

I live in my medium wash jeans that look like they could be plucked out of the '90s, but pretty soon you'll be finding me wearing darker washes. Sleek, polished, and a breath of fresh air in the world of jeans, this is the denim trend to buy in 2022.

4. SKIN-BARING EVERYTHING

There's no denying, it—skin-baring pieces get more ubiquitous by the season. Whether in the form of major cutouts or a cool bra top, there are so many ways to approach the trend.

5. VACATIONWEAR

Ready for a vacation? Same. When I pull the trigger and book a getaway in the year ahead, I'll have no shortage of cool things to pack in my suitcase and neither will you. Tropical prints and beachwear were top of mind for designers and the OOO aesthetic will be big.

6. LUXE STAPLES

Quality over quantity has always been my shopping mantra and it's also how many fashion people are curating their closets right now. Luxe staples are winning out, so look for expertly-crafted pieces to buy now and wear forever.

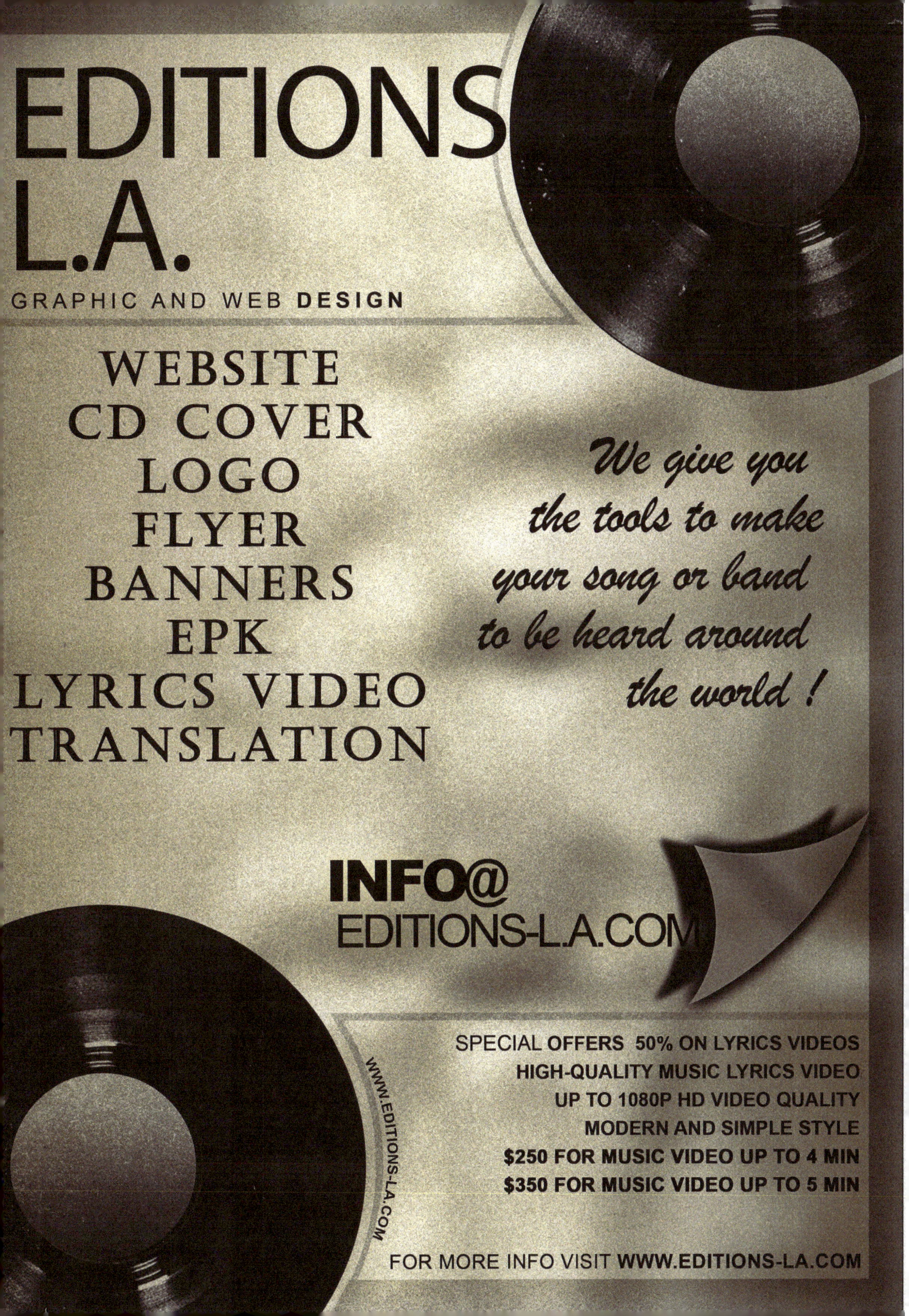

EDITIONS L.A.

GRAPHIC AND WEB DESIGN

WEBSITE
CD COVER
LOGO
FLYER
BANNERS
EPK
LYRICS VIDEO
TRANSLATION

We give you the tools to make your song or band to be heard around the world !

INFO@ EDITIONS-L.A.COM

WWW.EDITIONS-LA.COM

SPECIAL OFFERS 50% ON LYRICS VIDEOS
HIGH-QUALITY MUSIC LYRICS VIDEO
UP TO 1080P HD VIDEO QUALITY
MODERN AND SIMPLE STYLE
$250 FOR MUSIC VIDEO UP TO 4 MIN
$350 FOR MUSIC VIDEO UP TO 5 MIN

FOR MORE INFO VISIT WWW.EDITIONS-LA.COM

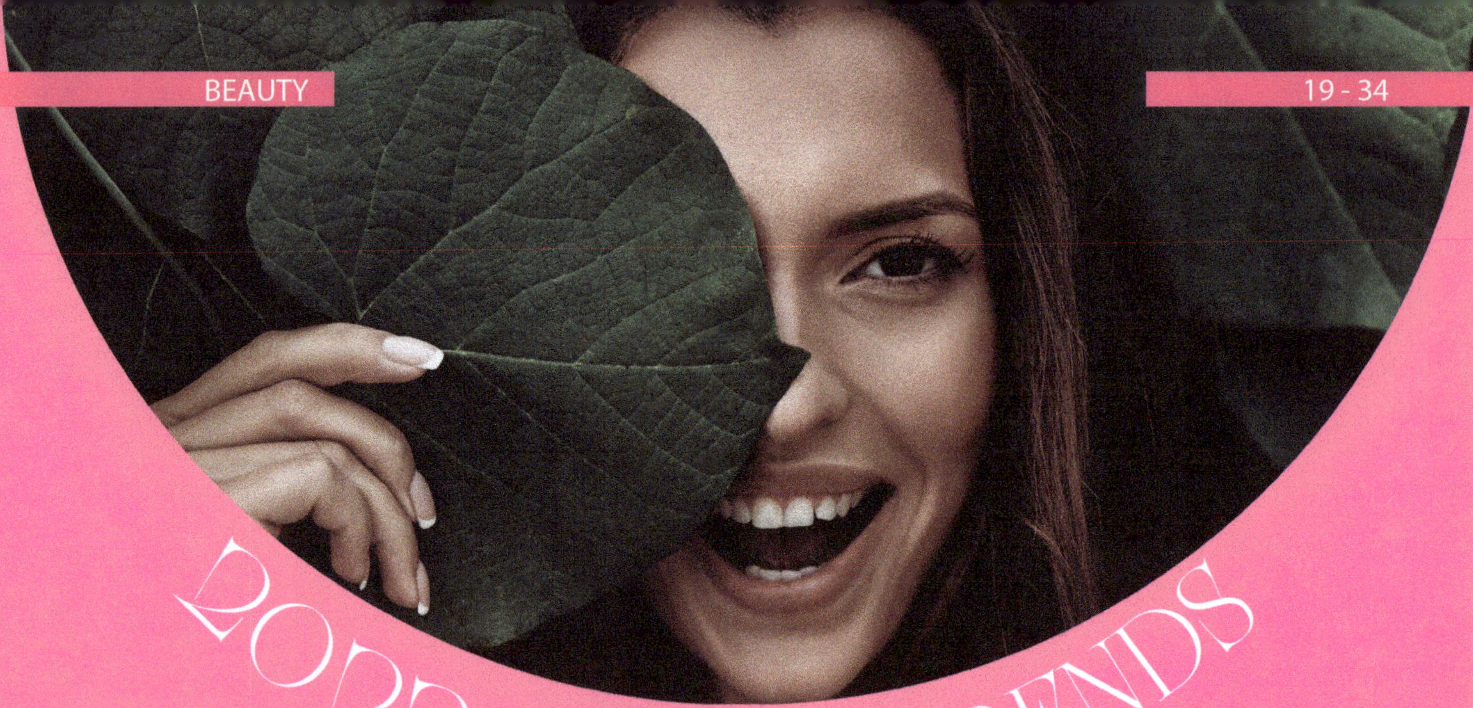

BEAUTY | 19 - 34

2022 BEAUTY TRENDS

LET'S GET BACK TO OUR ANCESTORS

BEAUTY ROUTINES

WE ARE PREDICTING WILL BE EVERYWHERE IN 2022.

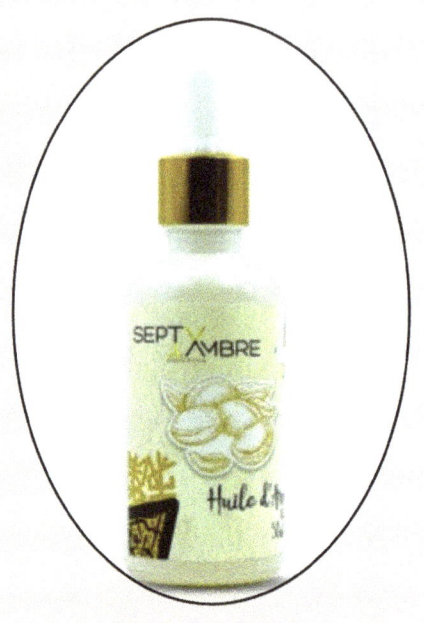

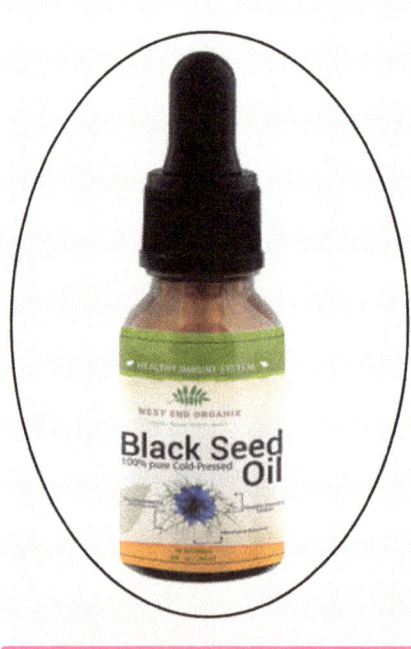

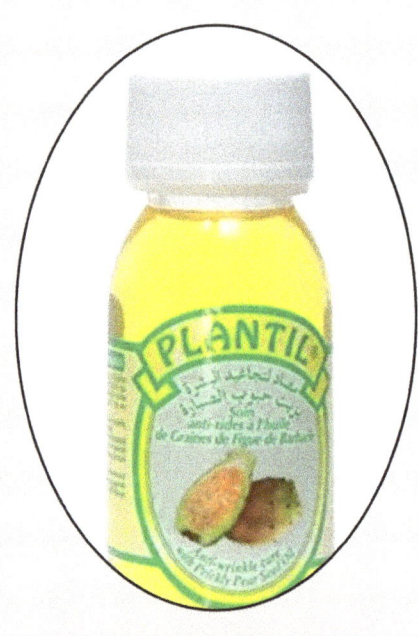

ARGAN OIL
www.SoinsMillenaires.com
@Soins_Millenaires

BLACK SEED OIL
www.WestEndOrganix.com
@WestEndOrganix

PRICKLY PEAR OIL
www.SoinsMillenaires.com
@Soins_Millenaires

VISIT OUR WEBSITE

BEAUTY TRENDS 2022

Natural oils, such as coconut oil, shea butter oil, and olive oil, have been used for skin care and hair care for centuries. Generation after generation have touted them for various moisturizing, protective, and antibacterial qualities. With the growth of the modern cosmetic and wellness industries, these deceptively simple substances have often been overlooked, but they've had a bit of a resurgence in the public eye over the last decade, as people strive to find additive-free, affordable, and effective products.

1. BLACK SEED OIL

Used cosmetically or topically in general, Black Cumin Seed Oil is reputed to effectively address fungal infections, yeast, and mold with its anti-fungal properties. Its antioxidant activity is known to promote the skin's elimination of harmful free radicals, thus diminishing the appearance of wrinkles, fine lines, dark spots, and other blemishes, thereby exhibiting a rejuvenating and revitalizing effect.

2. ARGAN OIL

Argan oil is a popular skincare oil that can help with skin barrier repair. Studies suggest that it has anti-inflammatory and wound-healing effects.
Topical application has also been shown to have an anti-aging effect on skin by improving skin elasticity

3. PRICKLY PEAR OIL

Prickly Pear Seed Oil is ideal for mature skin due to its exceptional hydrating and illuminating ability, but because it also has a comedogenic rating of 0 out of 5 (meaning it should not clog pores), it is effective with combination skin or those who struggle with acne too. For those wanting to tackle the signs of ageing before they happen, Prickly Pear Seed Oil is a must, particularly if toxin-free, natural skincare is important.

4. COCONUT OIL

Coconut oil is easily absorbed into the skin and is known to have many health benefits, including those from vitamins E and K, as well as its antifungal and antibacterial properties. The one big exception? Along with cocoa butter, coconut oil is likely to cause breakouts. "In general, coconut oil is a great option for almost everybody, except if you have oily skin and you're acne prone, I would not use it on the face," Katta says. In a study published in the journal Dermatitis, researchers found coconut oil was better than olive oil at moisturizing skin when used in a carrier. Remember to look for cold-pressed, unrefined coconut oil for your face or skin care.

5. TEA TREE OIL

Many natural oils can actually make acne worse, but not tea tree oil. The antimicrobial properties in tea tree oil help disinfect your pores while also reducing swelling and inflammation. A little goes a long way, though. Dab any area with a cotton swab dipped in a bit of tea tree oil

6. PEPPERMINT OIL

This herb is a mix between watermint and spearmint. The oils from peppermint leaves can have anti-inflammatory and antifungal properties, making it a good topical oil to alleviate skin conditions that produce itching.

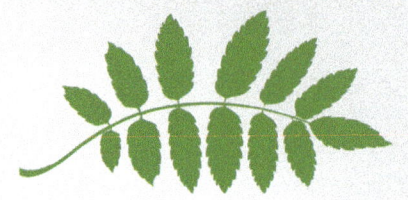

WEST END ORGANIX

Ageless Beauty, Organic Health

BLACK SEED OIL

HEALTHY IMMUNE SYSTEM
INFLAMMATORY RESPONSE

www.westendorganix.com

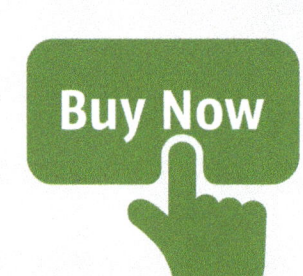

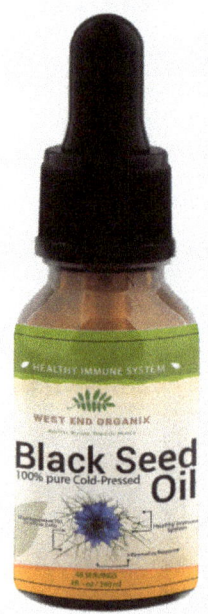

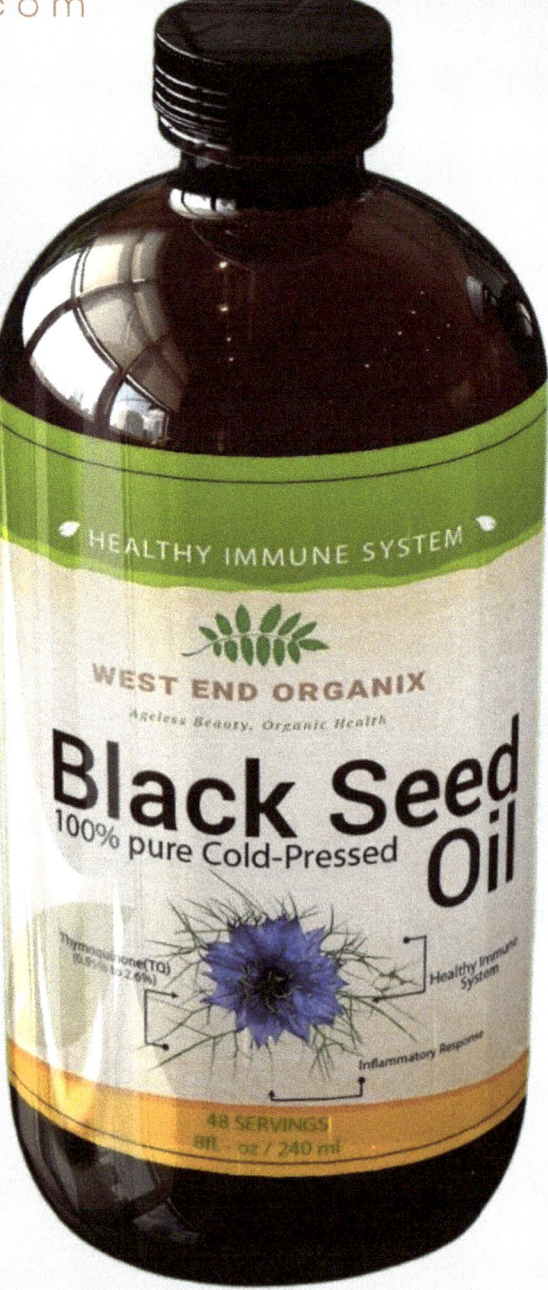

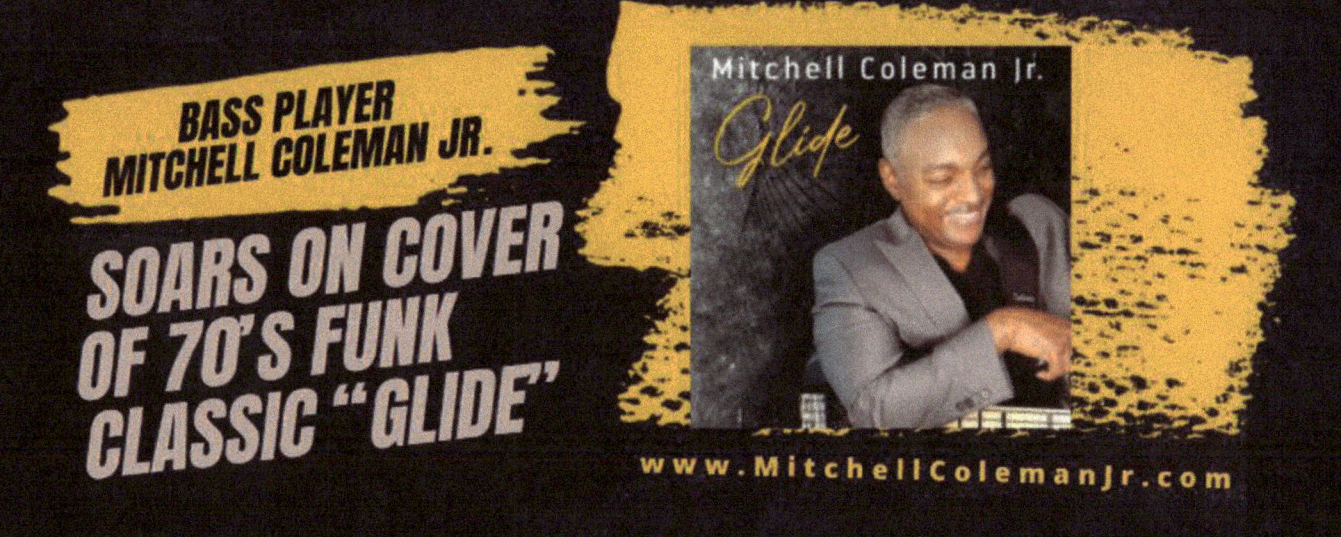

BASS PLAYER MITCHELL COLEMAN JR. SOARS ON COVER OF 70'S FUNK CLASSIC "GLIDE"

In a recording career that began in 2015 with his debut CD, Soul Searching, bassist Mitchell Coleman Jr. has been staking his claim as the new face of bass in your face FUNK. He is seriously throwing down the gauntlet with his latest single, *"Glide,"* a feel-good cover of the 1979 Funk classic originated by the band Pleasure. Where Portland-based Pleasure's original version (penned by the band's bassist Nathaniel Phillips w/ vocalist/percussionist Bruce Smith) was a tightly wound tapestry of Funk-Jazz, Mitchell Coleman Jr.'s take invites err'body to the skate party without skimping on 1 oz. of The Funk.

"The song just called out to me one morning," Coleman shares of his inspiration to boldly rerecord the Funk nugget.

"Glide" is one of those bucket list songs for bass players. Once you can play it, you know you're officially in the game. It took me a good minute to get this one under my thumb…`cuz Nate slid some serious stuff up in there! I would love to talk to him about that one day… I didn't want to mess with it too much. Just add a lil' of that Sylk Sonic skating flava. And lyrically, 'Glide' fits this time to a 'T.' There's just so many things we are all trying to get over and 'glide' on by…"

Coleman co-produced and worked closely with producer Michael B. Sutton and arranger Hiroshi Upshur, to give it a looser more universal appeal for listeners today as well as Funk connoisseurs who surely remember it from back in the day. Fernando Harkless also contributed via the spicy horn licks that he came up with and played in layers over the track.
The joyous result is a mighty good time for the head, heart and feets of all!

"Glide" is the lead-off single of Mitchell Coleman Jr.'s forthcoming third album which he is dedicating to the memory of his mother, Mary Ruth Coleman, who passed away two years ago. The working title for this project: Dedication).

In the meantime, *"Glide"* is dedicated to everyone around the world that likes to PARTY HEARTY in the face of today's relentless adversities.

"It's a tight groove," Coleman concludes, *"plus it highlights me as a bass player."*

Join Mitchell Coleman Jr. and get in touch to learn more about him:
http://www.mitchellcolemanjr.com/
For more information, follow: https://www.facebook.com/Mitchellcolemanjrofficialfanpage
https://www.instagram.com/Mitchellcolemanjr
http://www.thesoundofla.com

TOP INDIE ARTISTS

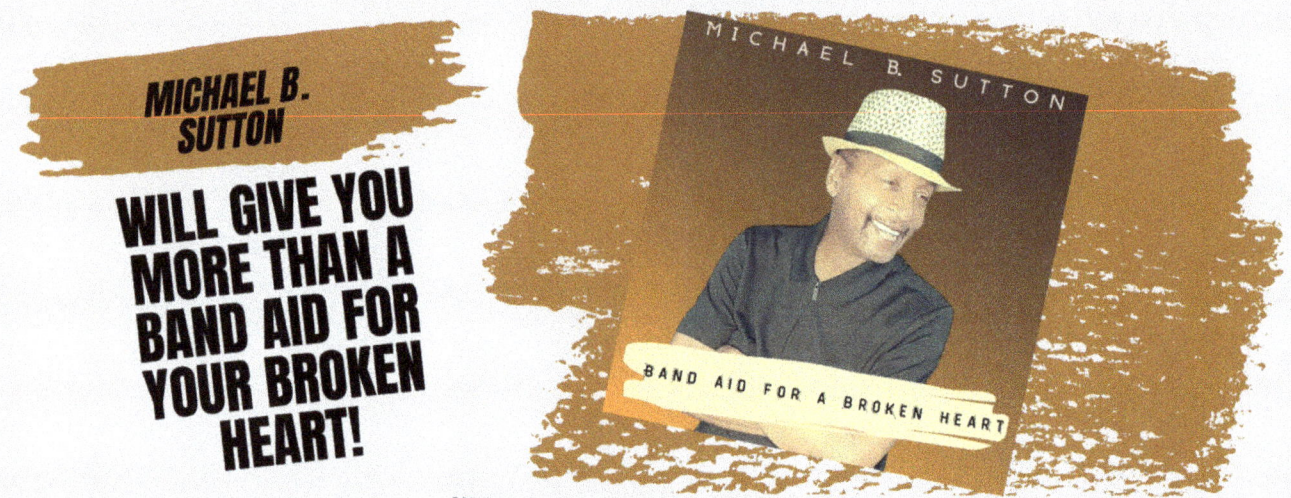

MICHAEL B. SUTTON
WILL GIVE YOU MORE THAN A BAND AID FOR YOUR BROKEN HEART!

WWW.THESOUNDOFLA.COM/MICHAELBSUTTON

C.E.O. at The Sound of L.A. and veteran Motown music producer MICHAEL B SUTTON has yet set out to begin this year with a crisp new sound that is about to mend all broken hearts. Thought of by many as one of the guides in the music industry, the LA-based singer and songwriter blends a sound of R&B and soul with his lyrical intimacy, attractive production, and organic rhythms on **his new single "Band Aid For A Broken Heart," (Download now exclusively on www.thesoundofla.com – Out on all digital platforms January 21st, 2022)**

"Band Aid For A Broken Heart" comes in with its elegant production and well-crafted lyrics written by Michael himself. The song speaks entirely about forgetting all that happened in the past and

Michael B Sutton is mending your heart for the new has come. Up-and-coming with a remedy more than the band aid itself, the prodigy promises an absolute healing for your pain that is about to last you till the end.
While we learn to take the driver's seat in many occurrences in our lives, Michael's latest track brings a change of view around us that opens new paths and reminds you that you don't have to be alone through everything. Usually, there is someone ready to offer a band aid for every broken piece that needs to be restored.
His new single invites us to be to be excited to be alive as we relive the feeling of being loved once again.

For over four decades in the music industry, Michael B Sutton has been well known for his personal nature, his honesty, integrity, professionalism, and attention to detail.
Having worked with some of the most celebrated acts of this century, including; Michael Jackson, Stevie Wonder, Thelma Houston, Diana Ross, Smokey Robinson, and more, Michael has proved to be one of the best producers and songwriters that has helped many artists on the way to stardom.
Whether he's only playing the piano, producing the sound, writing, or just singing vocals, he has proven to

Join Michael B. Sutton and get in touch to learn more about him:
Find Michael B Sutton & The Sound of L.A online;
https://www.thesoundofla.com

Apple Music: https://music.apple.com/de/artist/michael-b-sutton/6130621?l=en

Spotify: https://open.spotify.com/artist/7HXwMohQTjKQqjULUkd6kU?si=4-SWdDdjSGCdV02akZp3PQ

Pump it up Magazine / 23 - 32

Are you a songwriter or composer struggling to protect your work and releases?
Well Bernie Capodici has done all the work for you in his new book
"Modern Recording Artist Handbook, How To Guide Simplified"

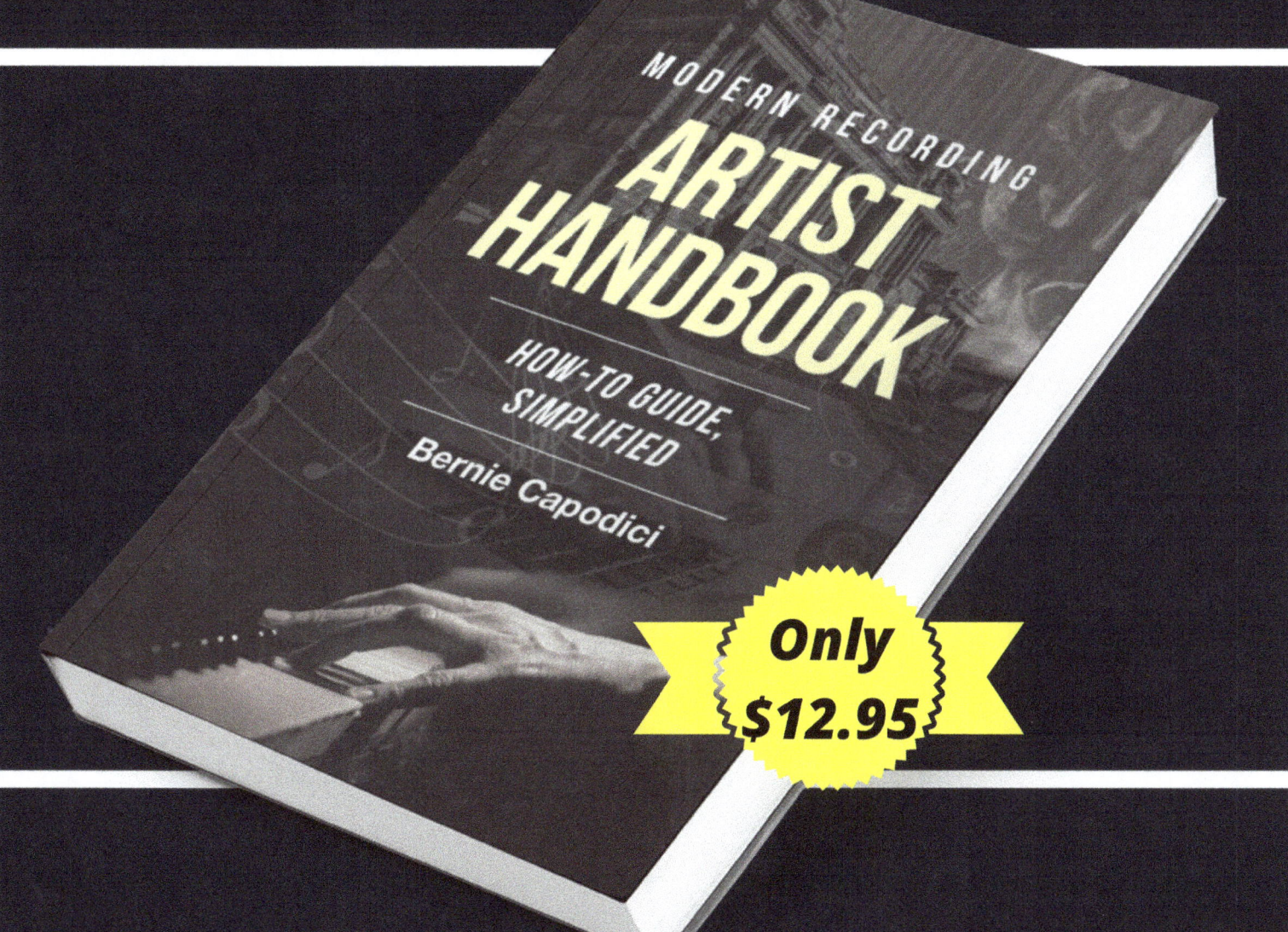

Only $12.95

MUST READ FOR INDEPENDENT ARTISTS

amazon   BARNES & NOBLE

KINDLE $9.99 - HARDCOVER $22.95 - PAPERBACK $12.95

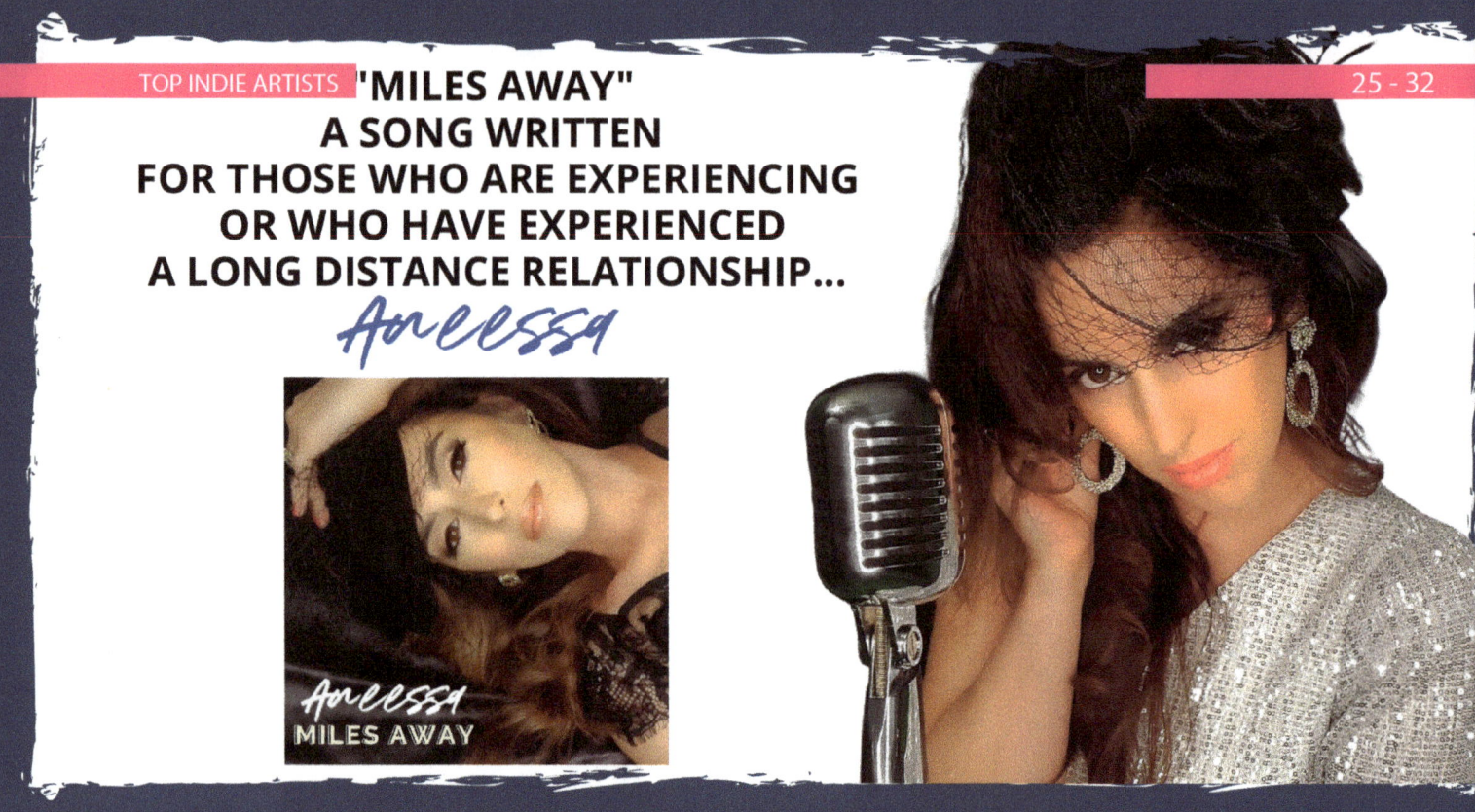

Married to veteran Motown LA producer Michael B Sutton, who also doubles as her producer, is sensational artist ANEESSA, a clear definition of the modern-day Songbird.

Hailing from Saint-Étienne in East-central France, Aneessa has had the opportunity to live in different cities around the world and experience different sounds and cultures. Her passion for music developed strongly as she explored life's various possibilities. She started performing while at a younger age and eventually took the dance music scene in Asia and Europe.

At this moment in life, she went by Anya Rose and Lady Aneessa.

Currently residing in LA, California, Aneessa has in the past years released music that is not only refreshing to the ears but also diverse in content. Her rich discography is a hiding place for so many music lovers, with her songs being widely streamed across major music streaming platforms in all parts of the world.

Inspired initially by international pop icon Madonna, Aneessa has always used her side time to make jazz, soul, and pop covers to some of her favorite Madonna tracks. Her recent release "Miles Away," released for now exclusively on her website, dropped as one of her popular Madonna song covers that she recorded this time with a neat touch of smooth jazz/pop.

The song was initially written by Madonna as a clear definition of how being in a long-distance relationship can raise so many untapped feelings.

Aneessa turned Madonna's old song into real-time gold that can be enjoyed by anyone going through a similar situation in life. Whatever distance is between you and your loved ones,

Miles Away cover by Aneessa is the song that is going to call you back to a place of comfort. She made a perfect cover song that features dreamy smooth jazz that will leave you asking for more.

The feeling of being away from your loved ones can raise a lot of mixed emotions and questions. Most people usually run to the internet and try to search for answers there. Even though everyone has a style in which they handle such emotional times, one common factor that is similar in all situations is the miles between the two of you.

Aneessa's Miles Away cover is one track that will lead you on a streak of understanding how to handle such emotions with its breathtaking production.

Find Aneessa on social media @AneessaMusic and Website ww.Aneessa.com
Label: The Sound of L.A https://www.thesoundofla.com

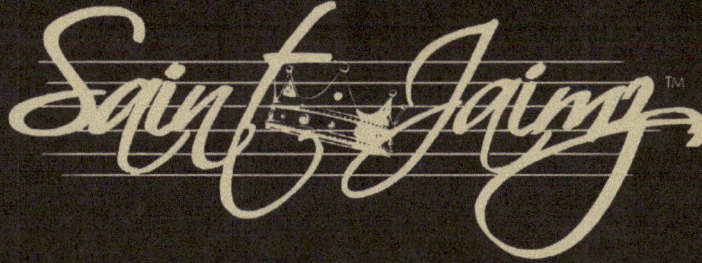

REVIVING THE ICONIC SOUND OF 90'S R&B

"THROWBACK, THE COVERS" VOL.1
A COMPILATION OF THE MOST TIMELESS 90'S R&B TRACKS

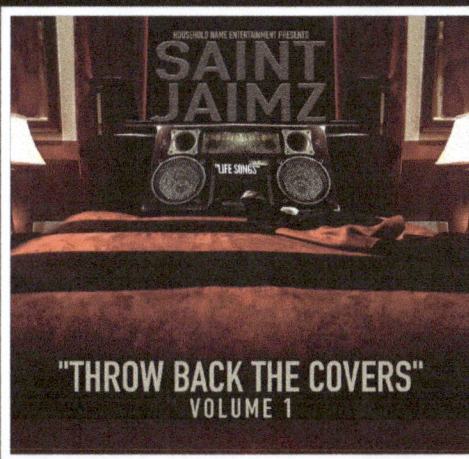

"THROW BACK THE COVERS"
VOLUME 1

www.SaintJaimz.com

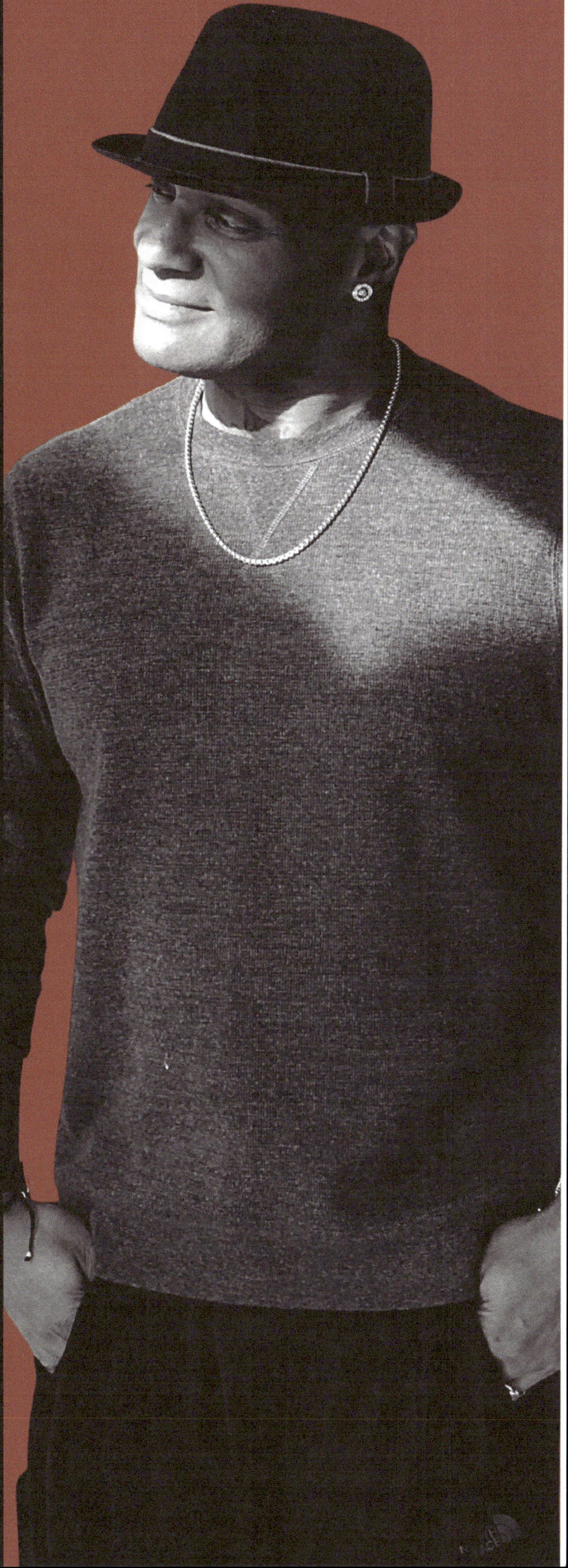

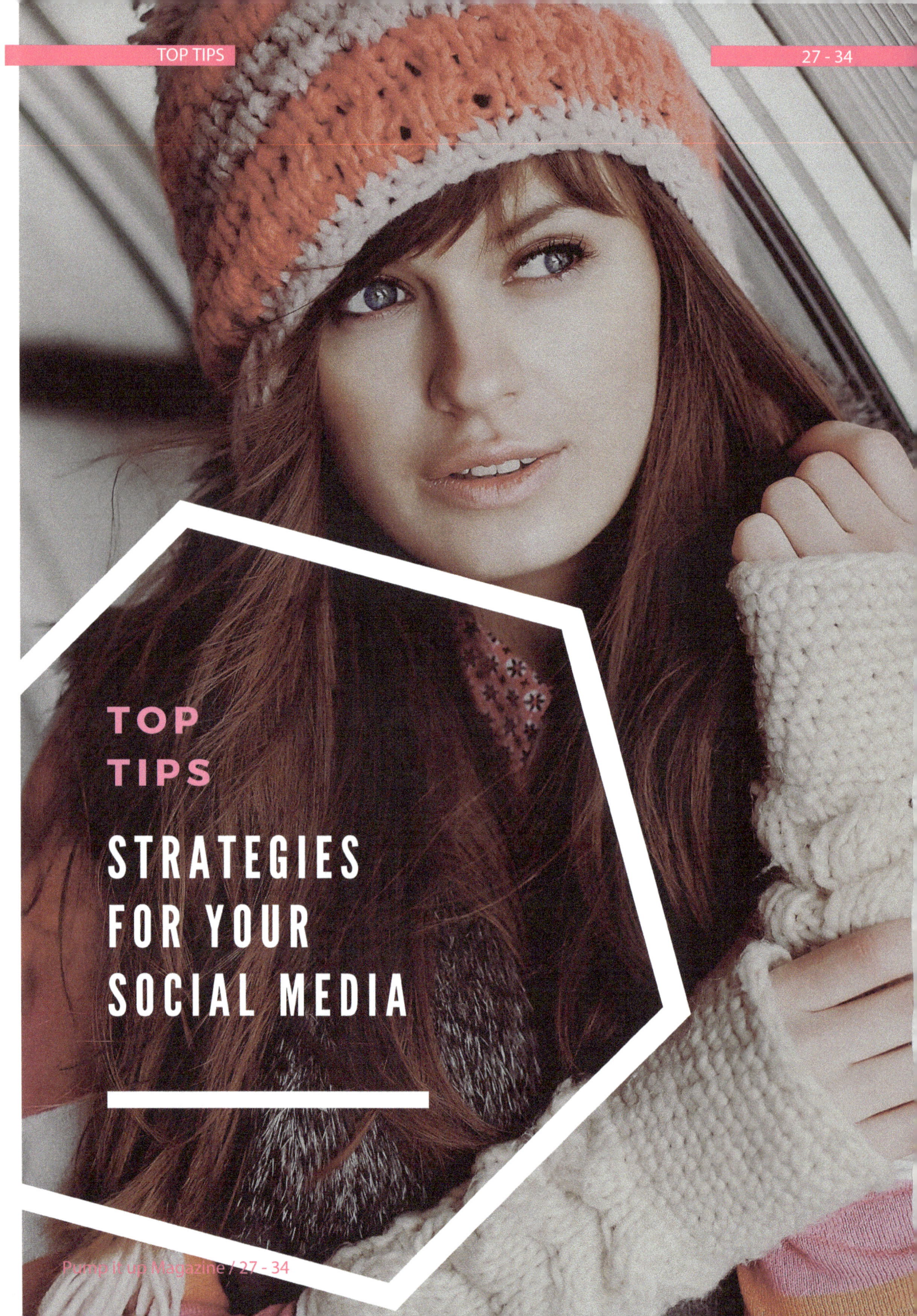

TOP TIPS

STRATEGIES FOR YOUR SOCIAL MEDIA

MUSICIAN SOCIAL MEDIA STRATEGIES FOR FACEBOOK, TWITTER, AND OTHER WEBSITES

There are do's and don't for using social media effectively, and that applies to musicians, too. Here's some basic advice to get the most out of social media as a hip hop artist, DJ, folk artist, or any other type of independent musician.

1. KEEP YOUR CONTENT VARIED

From a user's perspective, nothing is more boring (and eventually, annoying) than seeing repetitive posts over and over. You'll get more followers by mixing up your content to contain all sorts of material. Don't just blast your followers with requests for likes or retweets – give back! Upload videos, share photos, make creative use of hashtags, offer giveaways, share sneak peeks, discuss albums or equipment you enjoy, and don't forget to interact with your fans.truly unique about you, your artistry, and your story, and build out your brand identity from there.

2. DON'T POST TOO OFTEN – OR TOO LITTLE.

Different sources give different recommendations for the optimal posting frequency depending on factors like which website or app you're using and how many followers you have. Generally speaking, two posts per day is recommended for artists with large followings (10,000 or more), while a lower posting frequency is typically advised for musicians with smaller followings. Planetary Group can help you find an effective social media strategy for maximizing your visibility and outreach to listeners.

3. OFFER REWARDS FOR FANS

Who doesn't love being rewarded? You can make free downloads available to fans, or offer other simple, low-cost treats and exclusives, in exchange for liking your page or sharing a certain hashtag.

4. GET CREATIVE WITH INTERACTIVE FEATURES

Artists often fixate on the "media" aspect of social media and forget about the "social" part; but the beauty of social media is that it creates a two-way street. Not only can you share content with fans, they can share content with you – which also happens to be a great (and cost-free) way to make an impression and forge a connection. For example, you can invite fans to submit their art, upload videos, or simply share their opinions.

5. USE A PERSONAL TONE.

You're not the spokesperson for a multi-national corporation, so you shouldn't write like one on Facebook (or, for that matter, on any other social media site you're using). While you should definitely give your posts a once-over for basic grammar and readability, you should write like you speak so that your content has a genuine tone.

Facebook – 1.86 billion users - YouTube– 1.3 billion users - Instagram – 600 million monthly active users - Tumblr – 550 million monthly active users - LinkedIn – 467 million users - Twitter – 319 million monthly active users - Snapchat – 301 million monthly active users - SoundCloud – 175 million monthly listeners (40 million registered users) - Pinterest – 150 million monthly active users - Google+ – 111 million active users - Spotify – 50 million paid users (over 30 million tracks) - Last.fm – 44 million users (over 12 million tracks) - Musical.ly – 40 million monthly active users - Periscope – 10 million active users - ReverbNation – 3.8 million users - Bandcamp– Approximately 350,000 artists - Twitmusic – Over 50,000 registered artists

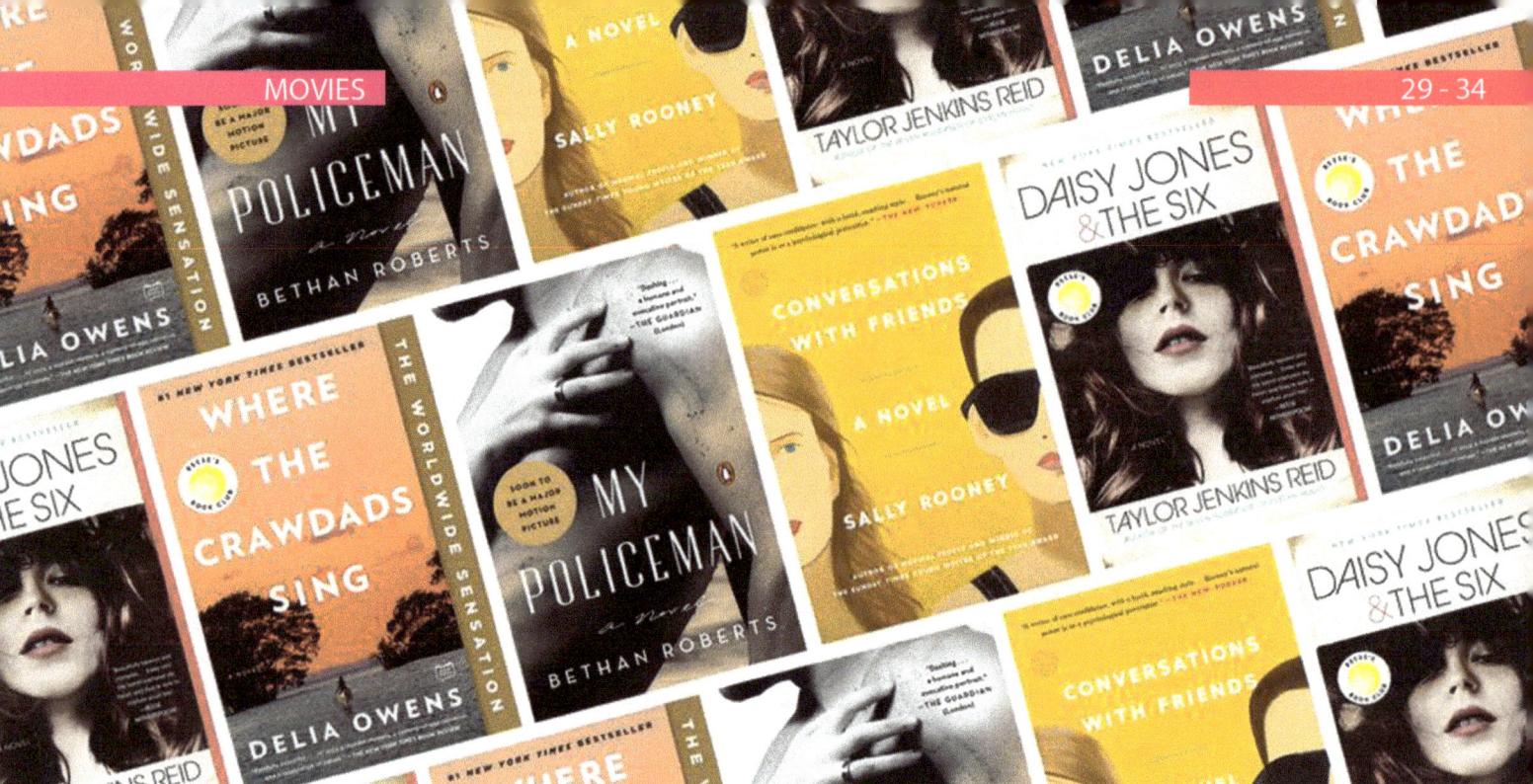

This past year has been packed with high-profile book adaptations, including sci-fi epic Dune, Jane Campion's neo-Western The Power of the Dog, and Lady Gaga-fronted crime thriller House of Gucci. So far, 2022's release slate is brimming with promising adaptations sprawling across a variety of genres, ranging from beloved classics (Persuasion) to psychothrillers (Deep Water) and romances (My Policeman).

In preparation for a year stuffed with film and TV adaptations, we've rounded up literary adaptations we're excited to see grace our screens.

1. PERSUASION

Jane Austen's novels have been translated to the screen for as long as we can remember, and they've increasingly received modernized interpretations (see: Clueless and Emma.).

This year, Netflix will retell this Regency era-set classic with a "modern, witty approach." Dakota Johnson will play Anne Elliot, the 27-year-old unmarried protagonist who reconnects with Captain Frederick Wentworth, a dashing and now-wealthy naval officer whose marriage proposal she turned down eight years before.

2. MY POLICEMAN

Bethan Roberts' 2012 novel centers on a heartbreaking love triangle between a police officer named Tom Burgess, his wife Marion, and a man named Patrick in 1950s Brighton, England. Set in a time when homosexuality was still illegal in Britain, Tom knows it would be "safer" for him to marry Marion than to be in a relationship with Patrick, so Marion and Patrick decide to begin sharing Tom, which ultimately proves to be destructive. On track to steal Hollywood's heart, Harry Styles will lead as the titular policeman. Opposite him will star The Crown's Emma Corrin and David Dawson, and the film is expected to land on Amazon later in 2022.

3. BLONDE

A lot has been said, written, and filmed about Marilyn Monroe over the years, and yet again, a biopic about the star will be released after almost 10 years in the making. Blonde is a 700-page, Pulitzer Prize-nominated novel by Joyce Carol Oates that tells a fictionalized account of Marilyn Monroe's private life. Ana de Armas will star as the Hollywood icon, and it'll feature a score from Nick Cave & Warren Ellis. While the film hasn't received an official date yet from Netflix, dig into the enormous book or watch Michelle Williams' underrated performance in My Week with Marilyn in the meantime.

MOVIES

4. THE NIGHTINGALE
Set against the backdrop of World War II, Kristin Hannah's novel tells the story of two sisters coming of age in France as they struggle to survive the German occupation. The story is inspired by the women of the French resistance who aided downed Allied soldiers in escaping Nazi-occupied territory and helped hide Jewish children. Actress-turned-director Mélanie Laurent will helm the adaptation based on a script by Dana Stevens. With real-life sisters Dakota and Elle Fanning starring, this will mark the first time the duo will play sisters on screen.

5. KILLERS OF THE FLOWER MOON: THE OSAGE MURDERS AND THE BIRTH OF THE FBI
A Western crime drama, David Grann's nonfiction book Killers of the Flower Moon: The Osage Murders and the Birth of the FBI investigates a series of murders of the Osage people in Osage county, Oklahoma that took place in the early 1920s after valuable oil was found on their land. The murders sparked a major investigation from the newly-formed FBI. Martin Scorsese's follow-up to The Irishman and first film with Apple TV+ will star a myriad of some of the best working actors, including Jesse Plemons, Leonardo DiCaprio, Lily Gladstone, Brendan Fraser, and Robert De Niro. Production wrapped last fall, so we can hope to see the film receive a 2022 release.

6. DEEP WATER
Patricia Highsmith has long been an inspiration for filmmakers, with her work serving as the source material for films including Purple Noon, The Talented Mr. Ripley, and Carol. Deep Water centers on Vic and Melinda Van Allen's loveless marriage as the couple begin to play mind games that turn deadly after their marriage crumbles. Former real-life partners Ben Affleck and Ana de Armas will star in the erotic psychological thriller. While it was originally slated to be released in theaters on Jan. 14, 2022, it will now stream on Hulu at a still-undisclosed date.

7. THE WONDER
A Western crime drama, David Grann's nonfiction book Killers of the Flower Moon: The Osage Murders and the Birth of the FBI investigates a series of murders of the Osage people in Osage county, Oklahoma that took place in the early 1920s after valuable oil was found on their land. The murders sparked a major investigation from the newly-formed FBI. Martin Scorsese's follow-up to The Irishman and first film with Apple TV+ will star a myriad of some of the best working actors, including Jesse Plemons, Leonardo DiCaprio, Lily Gladstone, Brendan Fraser, and Robert De Niro.

8. WHITE NOISE
Don Delillo's 1985 postmodern classic follows a couple, Jack Gladney and his fourth wife, Babette, and their four children as they find themselves at the center of an environmental disaster in their small Midwestern town. As part of a recent deal to produce films for Netflix, writer-director Noah Baumbach will reunite with frequent collaborators Greta Gerwig (who is also his partner) and Adam Driver, who will star in the lead roles. Jodie Turner-Smith, André 3000, Raffey Cassidy, Don Cheadle, Alessandro Nivola, and his children, Sam and May Nivola, will also star.

9. THREE WOMEN
Lisa Taddeo's debut nonfiction book is an intimate portrayal of female desire told from the true experiences of three American women who suffered for their sexual desires. There is Lina, a housewife in suburban Indiana who immerses herself in an affair with her high school sweetheart to escape from her passionless marriage. Sloane is an entrepreneur in the Northeast who has an open marriage with her husband Richard that becomes endangered after two strangers enter their lives. Lastly, there's Maggie, a student in North Dakota who must deal with the aftermath of accusing her teacher of inappropriate behavior. In the Showtime series, expected in fall 2022

THE STEPLADDER APPROACH
Helping children with anxiety through gradual exposure.

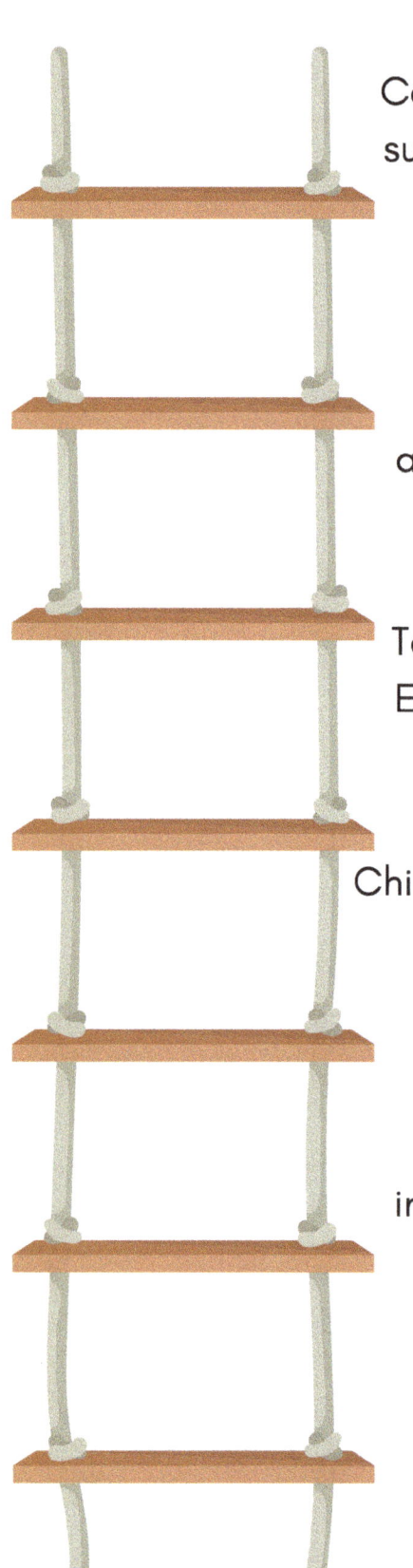

Collaboratively set a tangible end goal for success. What will the child be able to do when they are successful?

Set an end reward for motivation, and additional small incentives for each step.

Together, devise the first step to success. Ensure it is only mildly anxiety provoking.

Child can determine the level of anxiety each step brings, using a 10-point scale.

Continue devising steps together of increasing challenge and anxiety level to overcome the fear.

WORK TOGETHER

GIVE LOTS OF PRAISE

REWARDS AS INCENTIVES

HOW AMAZING IT IS ….WHEN I PAUSE AND REFLECT UPON….

…the mumblings of my mind…sometimes only a whisper….and sometimes amplified to an irritating roar…which causes my confusion….that which was so clear and normal …becomes distorted….causing me to stray away from my path…I enter a place where the light is dim….an ill chill of abandonment rushes in….as the mumblings of my mind becomes more prevalent….the sensation of being lost and abandoned….the sound of my mind mumblings become more distinct and precise….convincing me of the realities of the many images being thrust upon me….

The stomping boots of FEAR become louder and louder….as FEAR draws closer….intensifying my emotional response to the contorted vision of FEAR… Suddenly ….like a divine beacon….my darkness is illuminated…easing my anxiety and allowing me to pause and reflect….I become elated with a renewed sense of empowerment….I feel the presence of a POWER and LOVE …as my FEAR dissipates ….I once again feel connected to my soul and spirit….all those fearful things created from old memories begin to lose it's grasp upon me….I slowly breathe in HOW new air….pretending that each breath is a spoonful of necessary medicine….over and over I take deep breaths…and slowly let it leave carrying away all things which threaten me ….

MIND MUMBLINGS ….are now incorporated in my self defense medicine bag…for my awareness of MIND MUMBLINGS are now one of my various thermometers used to indicate my MIND MUMBLING thresholds…When I notice their presence…I can grab for my SELF DEFENSE MEDICAL BAG ….which also contain implements and medicine which I feel has been divinely design to nurture and care for me. How amazing it is ….when I pause and reflect upon the new discoveries which will come to me….to help me be …a better me….blessings and love ….
Temporary Activated Dust ….

Alan Laird

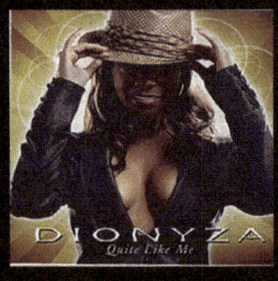

Pump it up MAGAZINE

RNB/SOUL ARTIST
DIONYZA

LISTEN TO HER ALBUM | QUITE LIKE ME
ON PUMP IT UP MAGAZINE RADIO

FROM 2PM TO 3PM (PST)

- QUITE LIKE ME -
DIONYZA
Quite Like Me
AVAILABLE EVERYWHERE

WWW.PUMPITUPMAGAZINE.COM

www.ingramcontent.com/pod-product-compliance
Lightning Source LLC
Chambersburg PA
CBHW051810010526
44118CB00024BA/2823